CANCER ETIOLOGY, DIAGNOSIS AND TREATMENTS

PSYCHONEUROCYBERNETIC CONQUEST OF CARCINOGENESIS AND CANCERS

CANCER ETIOLOGY, DIAGNOSIS AND TREATMENTS

Additional books in this series can be found on Nova's website under the Series tab.

Additional e-books in this series can be found on Nova's website under the e-book tab.

CANCER ETIOLOGY, DIAGNOSIS AND TREATMENTS

PSYCHONEUROCYBERNETIC CONQUEST OF CARCINOGENESIS AND CANCERS

RUDOLF KLIMEK

EDITOR

New York

Library of Congress Cataloging-in-Publication Data

ISBN: 978-1-63483-272-4

Library of Congress Control Number: 2015943823

Published by Nova Science Publishers, Inc. † New York

CONTENTS

PREFACE

"Medicine is one undivided human knowledge dealing with theoretical principles how to protect or restore health and simultaneously putting them into practice."

The most important value for a human being is life, which is transmitted by two gametes originating from each parent and it begins at the moment of conception, but the fetal maturity to independent life can be reached only in mother's womb. Physiologically, the life of an individual cell ends with its division into two cells of the same genetic type or as a result of dematerialization of its matter into energy needed for formation of biological structures, for what is already observed in embryo before its implantation in the uterus. The composition of blood is determined not only by the production of serum and blood cells, but also by the cells of blood vessels, which control and regulate its circulation in the whole body. The molecular biology has differentiated embryonic somatic cells and gametes from others, enabling their direct examination by nuclear magnetic resonance imaging and spectroscopy and also the possibility to distinguish cancer from pre-cancerous lesions or benign tumors. Also, similarly the evaluation of enzymes and hormone levels in maternal blood serves to successfully prevent early miscarriages and preterm deliveries by intramuscularly administrating adrenocorticotropic hormone. Fifty years ago, the treatment of mothers with neurohormonal insufficiency has eliminated fetal mortality, which had reached 80% even before treatment. Miscarriages, hemorrhages, infections and premature births are result of the damage of neurosecreting cells, which later manifest through a lack or a significant shortening of lactation, disturbance of menstruation up to its complete disappearance in 16% of cases, infertility, recurring inflammation, loss of hair, obesity, neurosis and precancerous stage of uterine cervix.

Quickly maturing cells of the immune system adapt their metabolism to the destruction of antigens, which induce their appearance. The continuous production of an enormous number of new bone marrow cells (4.10^{11} daily) is most susceptible to a change in genome, which is usually lethal but sometimes may result in autonomous cloning in the form of leukemia. During birth and rapidly thereafter microbes from the mother and the surrounding environment colonize the infant's gut. Humans coexist with a complement of prokaryotic symbionts that confer a variety of physiologic benefits, especially in the gastrointestinal tract where gut epithelia as a "super-organ" have a surface of 300-400 squared meters. Infants born by cesarean section are lacking a specific group of bacteria found in infants delivered vaginally, even if they were breastfed. With this in mind, it can have potentially lifelong effects on the child's health by increasing the risk of asthma, obesity, diabetes and cancer as man ages. Approximately 1.67 million women undergo this procedure every year in USA, but some caesarean deliveries are performed simply due by maternal request, what may incur several risks: neonatal depression, fetal injury respiratory distress, and breastfeeding complications or autoimmune diseases. According to the report of the third National U.S. Survey of Women's Childbearing experiences who gave birth in 2011-12, current cesarean section rate was of over 30% despite evidence that a rate of 5% to 10% would be optimal. Based on outcomes from thousandths non-medical indicated caesarean deliveries, such childbirth carries significant risk not only for the baby, but also are related to appearance of cervical cancer of mother. This cancer was diagnosed in 528000 people with 266000 deaths worldwide in 2012.

Cesarean section is still major abdominal surgery, which first of all has psycho-neuro-hormonal and immunological consequences with fundamental role of gut microbes in human health. The colonization of the gastrointestinal tract and vagina by symbiotic bacteria and cells of one's own immune system (lymphocytes, leukocytes, dendrites, macrophages, etc.) recognize the antigens of microbes. They create immunological antibodies strengthening the effectiveness of the neurohormonal and immunological processes of a person. Trials have demonstrated a rapid fall in the indicators of inflammatory states in vaginal smears and an improvement in the overall well-being of patients after administering the vaccine produced on the basis of symbiotic bacteria.

In 1974 Harald zur Hausen was unconvinced by the prevailing and popular belief that the herpes simplex virus cause cervical cancer, however between 1980-1982 his team has isolated first two human papilloma viruses (HPV) from genital warts and laryngeal papilloma as being causative factors also of cervical cancer. Beyond regulation by the HPV oncogene transcription there is evidence that the viral life cycle as well as HPV dependent tumor progression are rather determined by epigenetic mechanisms such as e.g., DNA methylation or even iatrogenic cesarean section. The fragmentation of the nuclear DNA by endonucleases (DNA-splitting enzyme) is a very early event of apoptosis and using DNA-methylation is critical marker for prognosis and the successful treatment of many cancers. High-risk HPV types are the primary necessary, but not sufficient carcinogenic factors of cervical, ano-genital and oral sites. Normal cells can be transformed by a variety of agents, such as chemicals, RNA or DNA viruses, radiation, and by transfer of DNA from tumor cells. In some cases introduction of a single viral gene is sufficient for transformation and may produce a single protein which can be very similar, or even identical, to normal cell components, but in transformed cells they are present in larger amounts. Neoplastic cells may show poorly regulated growth either by synthesizing this protein more rapidly or degrading it less rapidly, under conditions the limit normal cells' growth. Therefore, its accumulation is highly sensitive to factors that affect both processes. Spontaneous regression of carcinogenesis is commonly accompanied by humoral and cellular immune responses against specific antigens. HPV as the oldest virus still causes the warts today more often than at any time in its history. HPV and chlamydia infections, number of sex partners, the pill or smoking double risk of cervical cancer, while weakened immune and neurohormonal systems increases the risk after five years. Also the threatened pregnancy is linked with risk of cervical cancer. Women who have had 3 or more children have double risk of squamous cell cervical cancer as well as pregnancy before the age of 17 or over 25 among genetics-ethnic group with poorest social existence and chemical hazards at work.

The goal of the originated zygote *is the creation of the new being to uphold the species, but* the development of the first neoplastic cell only extends the cellular form of life without the possibility of autonomous existence. However, carcinogenesis cannot be eliminated, but illnesses which are caused by neoplastic cells can and should be treated, as they can be healed more often by direct fighting the pathogenic factors and indirectly strengthening the whole organism not only through neurohormonal therapy or immunopotentialisation with vaccines, but also using responsible information. For example, many obstetricians tread equally all so-called "at term fetuses," which on their view signifies 4-5 weeks. Therefore they often terminate pregnancy according to its calendar duration instead of the fetal developmental age, i.e., on which of these labor weeks the delivery has to occur. Prof. J.G.Schenker, president of International Academy of Human Reproduction summarized scientific contribution regarding the etiology of cancer and some new clinical approaches in clinical practice, saying e.g.: "Preterm birth is a major cause of neonatal mortality, responsible for 28% of neonatal death over all. One of the most important contribution to perinatology was the development of a new score for postnatal clinical assessment of fetal calendar maturity in newborn infants, which do not take into account weight and calendar fetal age, but refer directly to fetal maturity in the range of only 6-12 points. This publication encouraged the obstetricians performing birth-date prediction, which is possible with an accuracy of 3-4 days instead of weeks in order to prevent iatrogenic prematurity caused unnecessary induction of labor because false post-date.

In relation to cancer Rudi Klimek introduced a new concept regarding the etiology of cancer and its natural course with special attention to cancer of the reproductive track. At present, medical practice is based on evidence based medicine. Hopefully this interesting concept will be proven as it occurred with the Copernicans revolution – the heliocentric hypothesis."

Cancer cells grow in multicellular organisms, increasing dissipation of matter, information and energy in its environment, by which it kills normal cells destroying healthy tissues. Our book is an updated complementary volume to monograph *Explained Cause of Cancer* (Cracow 2013), as the result of our international uninterrupted cooperation since the first neurohormonal symposium entitled "Oxytocin and its analogues" (Cracow PTE 1964). Therefore, I desire to acknowledge the help and friendship received from so many P.T. Scientists who have contributed to this publication what can be seen from its contents and references, based upon multi years own experiences in conservative, surgical, thermo- and radiotherapy of neoplasms. They have summarized the public attitudes to cancer and infertility as well as supported the successive chapters of this book in relation to the historic discovery of natural psychoneurocybernetic cause of cancer, its mathematical interpretation, obstetrical prevention of human cancers and their therapy according to general, not only medical knowledge. Thenkfully everyman may understand the neoplastic diseases and the primary significance of own life style in the formation and progress of cancer along with importance of caring about the environment inhabited by people.

Prof.dr hab.med. Rudolf Klimek, Dr h.c.multi

LIST OF ABBREVIATIONS

ACTH	=	Adrenal Corticotropin Hormone
CIN	=	Cervical Intraepithelial Neoplasia
EDD	=	Expected Date of Delivery
FIGO	=	Federation International Gynecology Obstetrics
HPV	=	Human Papillomavirus

INTRODUCTION

Prof. Dr hab. eng. Ryszard Tadeusiewicz*, Dr h.c. mult.
Head of Automatic Control and Biomedical Engineering Chair and Director of Biocybernetics Laboratory in AGH University of Science and Technology, Poland

It is an honor to have been invited to write some word of introduction to this very interesting book, which is based on Video-document of International Multidisciplinary Symposium: Psychocybernetic conquest of carcinogenesis, (Poland Cracow 5th December 2013). Considered Symposium was very important and very interesting scientific event, located in Cracow Branch of Polish Academy of Science, therefore this book, which is main scientific result of such Symposium, can be seen as both important and interesting.

Let me begin form very general remark: The existence of societies dependent on legislative, executive and judiciary power is naturally regulated by information, but also the norms established by people cannot ignore the real natural rights, according to which the public interest is a priority. About 500 years ago, Nicolaus Copernicus from the University of Cracow (now Jagiellonian University) explained that the general belief that the Sun circulates around the Earth was based on an illusion. Then also in Cracow a hundred years ago, two main constituents of air were liquefied and it was simultaneously discovered, by famous scientists (physicists) Olszewski and Wróblewski. Next important discovery of scientists working in Cracow was disclosure, that the metabolism in animals resembles that of plants as

* e-mail: rtad@agh.edu.pl

confirmed by the hematin-like structure of hemoglobin, chlorophyll and lastly cytochrome S. Taking into account such examples we can consider now next discovery, discussed in presented book. It was revealed that cancers develop as a result of a natural and common phenomenon involving the self-organization of so-called dissipative structures from systems (cells) which are to be destroyed due to their thermodynamic insufficiency, cybernetically referred to as the emergence of negative entropy source, still is also quite astonishing, the source of entropy is life itself by coupled molecular processes increasing (positive source) and decreasing (negative source) its magnitude

Life, which is not human-made but passed from generation to generation for the maintenance of the species, is the highest good of a man. The life of a cell as the smallest independent biological unit is expressed by its spontaneous, reversible conversion of the matter and the energy of elementary particles along with the information on their state and their exchange with the environment as well as the ability to reproduce themselves. Multicellular organisms are composed of cells which psychoneurocybernetically match each other in terms of morphology (genetics), information and energy. The development of cybernetics makes it possible to distinguish between precancerous conditions and cancers, and thus enables conscious cancer prevention as well as initiation of causative instead of just only symptomatic treatment. The distinction between physiological and pathological cell metabolism has allowed to separate etiology from the analysis of morphologically and/or biochemically identifiable pathogenic changes underlying disease symptoms and ailments. The thermodynamic etiology of cancerogenesis, which provided new treatment alternatives in the case of standard management insufficiency or failure, is supported by the positive effects of hyperthermia therapy, which itself causes more damage to cancer cells than to healthy ones.

Cancers are only rarely genetically predeterminated, and the self-organization of a cell's genetic code is an effect, and not the cause of cancerogenesis. From a psychocybernetic point of view, biochemical and biophysical subcellular structures composed of multimolecular amino acids and nucleic acids, which, together or separately, are able to duplicate or reconstruct their fragments only together with the whole cell. Initially, cancers were diagnosed only in the final and usually fatal stage of the disease. Furthermore, it was discovered that cancers develop with unpredictable onset, course and recurrence in all body tissues and in people of all ages, that they come in different forms and eventually result in the destruction of the organism. Furthermore, it has been shown that the cause of cancer development may be associated with a number of different factors, which may cause the same morphological changes or where one of these factors may be implicated in the development of different forms of cancer. Radioactive radiation, for instance, causes different types of cancer in different body systems. However, before medicine starts to use technological knowledge to a greater extent, information, which besides matter and energy is an essential and equivalent component of reality, will play the key role in the protection of health. Even if a scientist is unable to find specific changes of matter and energy in the process of etiopathogenesis, there is information in every cause-effect relationship of structures and processes. Both structural and energy changes, which occur e.g., in a single cell, are in fact a change in information for the structures that surround this cell. The nature of new informational disease (informatonosis) lies in the source of harmful information that simultaneously relates to both an individual and a whole social group to which he or she belongs. The effectiveness of information is determined by the speed and range of its distribution via e.g., the Internet or other mass media, which considerably reduces the possibility to evaluate its accuracy, especially in terms of its source and the circumstances of its origins. The disease involves a number of social groups, and its incidence is affected by factors such as the predominance of negative news in the media, which results from attaching to them excessive significance due to their mediality. From the point of view of society, both terrorist attacks as well as the news concerning these attacks appear equally threatening. These sociological problems take on a new dimension once we begin to analyze the mentioned phenomena of social life in terms of medicine.

It should be understood that the word *cancer* refers to a chronic disease, although the term is frequently used in medicine to intimidate people and thus urge them to undergo preventive cancer screenings. Contrary to the prevailing customs, anticancer therapy should always be accompanied by the treatment of concomitant conditions as well as by the normalization of the patient's environment. Although tumors are also only rarely genetically predeterminated, all of them derive from genome self-organization. The universal mechanism of changes in the cellular genetic code is an effect and not the cause of carcinogenesis. The genetic identity of a human is created in the moment of conception, therefore pathologic course of pregnancy is associated with higher risk of cancer, and not only the cancer of the reproductive organs.

The beginning of the neoplastic illness is the appearance of a single cell, which, in order to sustain its diminishing metabolism, becomes a new entity (neoplasm) through the self-organization of the cellular genome, giving the cell a new identity. A characteristic of every neoplasm is its new genetic identity, stemming from the cellular DNA‘s self-organization as a result of the appearance of negative sources of phenomenological and informational entropy due to a decrease of metabolism. According to the second law of thermodynamics this generates new sources of positive entropy, which increases production of entropy both in the cell and in its environment, because a prerequisite for the existence of every cell is a positive sum of the entropy's increase in the system and its environment.

The state of the environment is determined by the number and the quality of blood and lymphatic vessels, whose endothelial cells perform an essential informational role in the metabolism of multi-cellular organisms. This means that the division of neoplastic cells as a fundamental characteristic of cellular existence is dependant upon the existing and emerging vessels in their environment. Neogenesis cannot exist without angiogenesis, i.e., processes dependant both upon the state of neoplastic cells and the endangered organism's own cells.

The symptoms of neoplastic illnesses are an effect of the influence of the dissipation of matter, information, and energy by neoplasitc cells upon the inner state of the sick, or only old, person, which forces prevention, prophylactics and treatment of neoplasm as an additional, but never the only reason for the loss and endangerment of human life. The symptoms and the illness caused by somatic neoplasms are linked by the neogenesis to psychoses and peoples‘ anti-human informatonosis. Neogenesis, in the light of the given by R. Klimek universal formula of reality $E \overset{i}{\rightleftharpoons} mc^2$, results from the possibility of exchanging the mass of the cell's useless organelles for the energy needed for the self-organization of the cellular genome of the cells which are in a dissipathogenic state, also called a pre-cancerous state.

REFERENCES

Czajkowsk, Krzysztof; Klimek Rudolf, Panikova Lubomira, Sikora Jerzy, Stencl Jan, Tholt Marian, Valent Michal, Ventruba Pavel: Obstetrical informatonosis - diagnosis and treatment.

Klimek, Rudolf: Formula $E \overset{i}{\rightleftharpoons} mc^2$ of the threefold material-informational-energetic universe: An Update.

Klimek, Rudolf, Joseph G Schenker: Gynecological prevention of iatrogenic carcinogenesis.

Szymański, Marek: Neovascularization and Neoangiogenesis in Differentiating Adnexal Lesions with Contrast-Enhanced Transvaginal Ultrasound.

In: Psychoneurocybernetic Conquest …
Editor: Rudolf Klimek
ISBN: 978-1-63483-272-4

Chapter 1

FORMULA OF THE THREEFOLD MATERIAL-INFORMATIONAL-ENERGETIC UNIVERSE: AN UPDATE

Rudolf Klimek*
Fertility Centre, Cracow, Poland

"In the beginning there was the word, and in it, life"
Old Testament

ABSTRACT

Man through the informational state of his "I" (Ego) defines his relationship to truth and good of his environment. The formula E $\underline{\leftarrow i \rightarrow}$ mc^2 helps in understanding the causal purposefulness of observed structures and processes in liaison with the causative role of information, which is inseparable linked with their mass and energy. The reality formula is the basis for all processes of life (including carcinogenesis) as a spontaneous mutual interchange of the matter, information and energy of elementary particles coupled with information about their state. Any body cell threatened with the end of its metabolism may self-organize in the form of cancer by increasing the dissipation of information, matter

* Corresponding author: Prof. Rudolf Klimek. Fertility Centre, Cracow, Pl.Szczepański 3, 31-011 Cracow, Poland. e-mail: mmklimek@cyfronet.pl, phone: +48601547436, fax: +48-12 4225684.

and energy in the multicellular organism. Once death occurs, the atoms of which the body is made fall apart into independent entities, but the person's past deeds leave behind accessible information about his unique life, which already began in the program of his zygote, and still exists in his informational legacy or in the social memory of it.

Keywords: Cancer, carcinogenesis, dissipative structures, entropy, human life, information, sources of generative entropy

INTRODUCTION

People are forming sentences in different languages, but their informational meaning depends on their common social environment. This is why it is important to understand the titular quote of this review article, especially "the word, and in it, life." A word is a particle of information which links the unbreakable material-energetic constituents of all living beings, including man, as the most highly organized multicellular organism due to his use of lingual information. This is not easy from a psycho-medical viewpoint if one also considers the biblical statement about humans: "before I created you in the mother's womb, I knew you" (Jr.1,5). Therefore when and where is the beginning of every material-energetic human existence which humans perceive with their senses? In response to this question in 1990 I published article, which I began with Karol Wojtyla's motto from 1972: "The journey through death towards life is a mystery. A mystery not entirely examined" [1]. At that time I understood the word "mystery" which unites faith and science, respectively both religious dogma and Heisenberg's uncertainty principle. After further years of research and life experiences due to the discovery of the thermodynamic cause of cancer in 1977 as well as the explanation of the concept of human death, I decided to interpret the statement of John Paul II: "The empty grave is the sign of man's eternal life" which he explained many times, as well as a quote from the encyclical Fides et Ratio "Behind a single word are hidden many meanings. At first one must more precisely determine its meaning. Moved by the desire to discover the final truth of his existence, man attempts to gain certain elements of universal knowledge, which help him understand and further realize himself." Which is why at the beginning I shall explain my understanding of the review's title before me theoretically and medically prove it with facts by describing the diagnosis and informational treatment of neoplasm diseases, as well as the socio-economical disease of social life called informatonosis.

A Zygote As a Unique Cell with a Unique Informational Identity

Every person is statistically determined biologically unity from the moment of the unification of two reproductive gametes with their unique identity [2-5]. Since in the XIX century Rudolf Virchow described the human construction as a multi-cellular structure, humans seek to find life also in individual unit-cellular forms, recognizing the ability of direct division, or an indirect transformation into other cells as a basic criterion of their existence. In view of this red blood cells (erythrocytes) should not be called cells, because they have neither nucleus nor other cellular structures (e.g., mitochondria, Golgi apparatus) and subsequently they cannot divide. Another type of human cells similar in this aspect are female (ova) and male (spermatozoa) reproductive gametes. Only after fertilization they create a true cell, unique compared to the cells of the father and mother, and capable of division into three types of clone cells. The first one is responsible for the creation of human with the ability to reproduce, the second are gametes, and the third, together with the mother, is responsible for the correct intrauterine development of the child, e.g., the cells of placenta existing until birth, when the tolerance of the mother's organism toward them ends. A person's genetic identity appears in the moment the gametes with different parental identities merge into a unique, new one creature. The biological importance of the zygote is demonstrated by the huge selection of millions of spermatozoa and hundreds of thousands of egg cells, from which only two gametes are going to be used at the moment of conception. The reason for the death of such a large number of cells in order to create one zygote does not seem to be accidental [6-9]. This is a statistically defined phenomenon in the shape of a realization of o human life as an inter-generational transfer of life between individuals, what depends also on the gametes of their grandparents. From the moment of fertilization the cells which developed from the zygotes ensure the maturation of a fetus which is able to pass on life through generative cells of its own and due to the simultaneously developing of pregnancy cells they condition the recreational health of the mother. The problem lies in the fact that one tries to separate the purely informational aspect (the perception of a personal "I") from the informational program of the whole material-energetic development of a person which is embedded in the zygote.

INFORMATIONAL ASPECTS OF THE TRIPLE-FORM BEING

In reality information describes the magnitude of the order of any system, i.e., its material and energetic constituents. By a scientific definition the system is any part separated from reality, and the rest of the world is called the environment [10, 11]. One cannot separate the name of the system or its environment from their triple form, which combines mass (m), energy (E), and information (i). In the search for universal laws describing the functioning of the universe, the material-informational-energetic formulation takes a special place, because it helps to understand the cause of observable occurrences (structures, processes) together with the influence of the environment, due to taking the causal effect of information into account. The sense of including information in the formula $E \underline{\leftarrow i \rightarrow} mc^2$ can be demonstrated by the behavior of a mass and an energy of water molecules in the unstable flow of a river, especially in mountainous rapids. The width and inclination of the riverbed constitutes important information for the mass and energy of the water molecules of the water flowing in a given unit of time. Information alone does not only describe a fact or an analysis of data, but is primarily responsible for the material-energetic relationship of elementary particles in both the system and its environment.

For a person information is a motivation for an act or idleness, depending on this person knowledge, which can be perceived as the role of the riverbed's informational role in the stream of the river. One can easily find matter and energy in an object, like a metal coin held in a hand. The imprint represents its monetary value, but does not describe all of the information contained within. However, in the other empty hand there is only information, in other words the concept of "nothing." It is enough to hold a material object containing kinetic or gravitational energy in one hand and nothing in the other to understand that both hands are linked by the difficult-to-understand information described by the word "nothing" in one hand, and information hidden in the material-energetic thing in the other hand, perceived by a number of quanta. This understanding of information only requires measure, similarly to the mass and energy, e.g., example a gram is a quantum of a ton, a centimeter of a meter, a second of an hour. The smallest unit of information describing all possible states of a system is a qubit.

Every matter-information-energy system (structure, process) in the universe contains in its cause information, as a programmed goal of its function, which is a desired and immediately afterwards created effect, in the cause-effect link of occurrences. The changes which happen during this process are always accompanied by the creation of useless entropy, the magnitude of which is also described using qubits. In medicine this allowed to understand the origin of ageing and cancer. Ageing is characterized by a gradual loss of an internal equilibrium and by a lessened ability for self-defense and self-regulation of the system in response to the environment action. It results in an increased of weariness, as a measure of entropy, the production of which is always greater than zero. This pertains to human consciousness, regardless of how we call it: ego, "I," a person or a name. For a long time thinking was attributed to the brain, as if that part of the body could function without the circulation of blood and breathing. Such, although not exactly the same, atoms make up the heart, lungs and brain, but in the field of nucleomagnetic imaging they all resonate differently depending on their environment and the inner state of the person, taking the psycho-emotional life, and even gender into account. So what is consciousness, which is felt by every person? The answer to this question is possible by defining the life itself as a spontaneous continuous exchange of matter and energy of elementary particles coupled with information about their state [4]. The word "spontaneity" without explaining its source, fulfills, in this definition, the role of one of many variables in mathematical-physical equations, or ones yet awaiting definition. Paraphrasing this statement one could think that in the beginning of the world there could not have been a scientifically defined concept of the word, but an unknown informational qubit in its core. This means that the Bible contained the information itself, written as the word, without the co-existence of its carrier, and in it the announced life, i.e., life *in statu nascendi* of humans and the universe. Etymologically "information" means the act of informing or the action of giving the form to the subject, thus realizing natural chance and development [5-8].

Generative Entropy

The concept of entropy is important because of its involvement in every material-energetic change, the more so the less organized it is. The appearance of mass in the moment of the experimental creation of the Higgs particle proves that entropy appears each time anew, and its value must be greater than zero for the system to function [9, 10]. More so, if in the system its production is reduced (physicists call this a negative source of entropy), the system may endure through an increase in entropy production in its environment through an increased dissipation of mass, information and energy.

According to the laws of thermodynamics a cell threatened with the end of its metabolism may extend its life in the form of a neoplasm cell by decreasing the production of its own entropy together with the increase of dissipation of information, mass and energy in the environment.

The basis for all irreversible life processes, including of course carcinogenesis, are the changes (d) in the production of entropy (diS) through time (dt) carrying the name of the generated entropy:

$$\frac{d_i S}{dt} \equiv \dot{S}_{gen},$$

for the existence of which its value must be greater than zero. In the end it is the sum of entropy increase of the system and environment, what is taken into account by the formula of reality E $\underline{\leftarrow i \rightarrow}$ mc^2, in which "i" stands also for the generative entropy of the system. This is why oncology prophylactics and treatment, apart from the ageing of the organism, must take into account other non-cancerous diseases which accompany the neoplastic one. In such a cellular change of life forms the only stable ones are the primary cellular states and the neoplasm formed from them, and the middle state of dysplasia is characterized by an increase in fluctuation of opposing metabolic processes.

Large fluctuations may destroy cells which are easily affected by the interaction with their surroundings, while small fluctuations may offer the chance of steering every system onto new metabolism paths. The basic property of neoplasm cells is not an acquired one, but their own trait in the form of their own unique, self-organizing under the influence of negative sources of entropy to keep the cellular metabolism by dissipating mass, information, and energy in the proximity of the neoplasm. It is this which allows for the creation of new identical cells according to the three-dimensional reality. The increased dissipation becomes a local sign of the beginning of an illness threatening the existence of the whole multi-cellular organism, which answers via neo angiogenesis, the widening of blood and lymphatic vessels in the area of the neoplasm, being a morphological effect of previous biophysical, biochemical and immunological changes.

The deciding factor for a neoplasm illness is the effectiveness of the immune system upon the individual cancer cells, the destruction of which by phagocytes can presently be imaged in real-time. Due to modern technology one may define the most endangered parts of the organism via magnetic resonance and spectroscopy. After the removal or even a reduction of neoplasm tissue, the use of hyperthermia adds to the classical surgical methods, which results in a lower possibility of acquiring the marginal tissue around the neoplasm one to guarantee oncologic sterility, which guarantees the removal of all neoplasm cancers in the way of eliminating germs. Finally, the modern thermodynamic method, (the surprise analysis) found a direct use to determine the characteristic changes of energetic nucleotide genes in cells undergoing carcinogenesis.

HUMAN LIFE WITH ITS OWN GENETIC IDENTITY

The objective existence of information as a background without a border from its environment – enables in consequence the understanding the informational identity of the human being and the possibility of knowing the moment of its emergence. The impossibility of determining the system's informational borders turns out to be non-coincidental, since every reproductive gametes contains a programmed potential morphologic-informational-energetic human life. The goal of the created zygote is to sustain the human species through the programmed development of the three coexisting cell groups (clones), of which two will co-create a new human being. These clones contain the informational component of the individual human lifespan, together with the psycho-emotional life-aspect.

Teleology seeks the goal (program or function) already in the cause of any event, and so the identity of every individual is determined already during the creation of the zygote, characterized by spontaneous mutual interchange of its elementary particles. In this spontaneity lies the ultimate cause of the universe, described in the Bible as the "word," which existed in the beginning before man began describing with his thoughts his environment and reality, to finally understand his own consciousness, his own "I" as an extra-material motivation of his life and actions thus defining his relationship towards existence, truth and good [12]. From the moment of death on, the atoms of the body of the deceased disintegrate into separate entities, but from the actions of the person the information about his social life remains, beginning in the program of the zygote he stemmed from, and still exists in human experiences or the memory of them. The identity of each individual, experienced as his own "I," is pure information, the only distinguishing, also informational carrier is his name, what, in my opinion, comes easiest, but is most difficult to maintain despite received titles and offices. The name is a result of reality, begun information in the moment of fertilization. The uniqueness of information is based on its ability to exist independently, as opposed to matter and energy, changes in which are accompanied by an increase in entropy, being a measure of order in every system, and as the opposite of information may serve as a plan for further order.

The Effectiveness of Information

An understanding of information stops being something unimaginable when through an analogy we relate it to the missing nucleic part of the human papillomavirus (HPV) inside its protein shell during prophylactic vaccination. Such a vaccine has been created (Gardasil, Silgard, Cervirax) against infections with this virus, which was rightfully awarded with the Nobel Prize [13-15]. In my opinion the HPV-DNA parts of the cancer cellular DNA play primary role in maintenance of the self-transformed cells. Cervical cancer is a clonal disease and for that reason the original HPV viral part of cell genome maybe a source of many HPV viruses appearing during material degradation of exfoliated cervical cancer-cells. Unfortunately, contrary to current knowledge, some researchers called Gardasil, Silard or Cervirax "the first and single vaccine against cervical cancer" instead of against a number of types of this virus [10, 16-20]. Not only do they continue to consciously lie to their patients, but even publicly explain this with the desire to increase sales. Two basic facts are omitted. Firstly, the HPV virus, in order to spread, utilizes the physiological fact of shedding epithelium cells of the vagina and mouth. Humans have through the ages worked out methods of reducing this viral infection in up to 80% of the cases. This is why the virus continually changes its protein shell, which the infected organism detects and fights. Secondly, an injection of such a vaccine under the epithelium is a transmission of two pieces of information: the viral infection has already gone through the epithelial defense barrier of the person, and, more importantly, there is a virus inside the vaccine which is actually not really there! Thus an excessive reaction, especially of a not completely healthy organism, can become the cause of the illness or even death of a person. In this way not the virus itself, but the false information about its existence often leads to court cases in favor of the deceived patients. This example should show the existence of causal information in reference to the most well known and most important information about the empty Jerusalem grave of Christ. It is well to use this statement, since according to John Paul II this empty grave is a "new uprising, new attest of faith, good deeds, love, justice, compassion" He repeatedly said that the church and the whole world waits, because "the hour of Christ's victory over death is the greatest hour of his deeds, when he killed death" In the words of saint Paul "Where sin occurs, there even more so spills compassion" (Rz.5,20). One should note that the words of the Pope refer not only to the personal, but also the social life of a person. According to John Paul II: "The need to think in categories of the whole, it is not about shallow empiricism, but one needs to reach beyond empirical data so that in one's search for truth one may find something absolute, final, fundamental... To days man seems to be always in danger by that which is of his own making." John Paul II not only discarded communism, but also criticized capitalism, because this social and economic system does nothing for moral awareness, because independently of declaration, it removes all values excepting ones measured by gain or economic growth. But he did point to the necessity of loving one's neighbor [3, 21]. It should be noted that truth itself is a potent medicine in informational diseases of social life, but not enough when it comes to the organization of anti-humanitarian activity of people who destroy social life not retreating before deadly dangers to people who do not share their views or deeds [22-26].

F. Collins called the nucleotide genetic code the language of God due to its universal reach [27]. Similarly, one may see God's gift of free will and the following of the Decalogue in the local formulation of the second law of thermodynamics saying that the negative source of entropy generates its positive source. This means that in the universe good always defeats evil because it is the informational equivalent of faith and hope. This happens because the natural laws work harmoniously and without the involvement of humans, who only interpret the universe more or less correctly and may disrupt it locally, but not globally. Already Leonardo da Vinci stated that nature does nothing in excess or with mistakes, while John Paul II added that: "modern man seems to be continually endangered by what is his own creation." This is why it's essential to form character of a person through education to not search for personal gain at the cost of human society, but to act according to a personal vision of the world [3, 21, 28]. The Holy Father taught the necessity of thinking in categories of the whole: "Between God and man – although each lives in his own world – there exists a unique mutual bond. In God there is the beginning of all things, in Him there lives the secret, and that creates His glory; it is man's purpose to examine truth via reason, and that is his dignity" [3]. God does not throw words into the wind, because His right, independent of whether man believes in Him or not, is based upon the natural laws he created before the truth contained within them could be discovered by men of science, which I have thermodynamically shown in "The Decalogue as a theological program of the Holy Trinity in the creation of the world," lectured in the year 2011 during the interdisciplinary session "Man and the Universe" to honor the discoverer of extra-solar galaxies by K. Rudnicki [6, 22, 26].

CONCLUSION

Man, as an individual part of society working and living due to free will defines his relationship with truth and good through the informational state of his "I" not only through action, but also through inaction towards his environment. He himself is shaped by his environment, for example the people who live in similar environments on earth and want to improve the world, which they can understand more and more now have similar character. Before concluding, I would like to quote a part of my consideration on the spiritual life of humans, published in 1990: "Nobody would ever consider to isolate reproductive cells from the wholeness of the organism, of which they are an integral part. Furthermore, they pass on all their traits to their progeny, therefore also morality, thoughts, and feelings. One simply should cast aside the absurd idea of where, in the egg cell or the sperm, one can localize the equivalent of the thought or morals of the children. According to medical thermodynamics it is enough to consider them as integral part of these cells. In the end function also determines the structure, but can these considerations also pertain to man's soul, a problem of not only believers. The relationship between the soul and the body, or vice-versa – still occupies a special place in philosophy. Nobody tries to localize the soul in reproductive cells because it is so tied together with the human being, and not with its separate parts. Saint Thomas held the spirituality of the person only in the 40th day of the pregnancy, and today this day is also recognized by orthodox Jews. The thing is it is impossible to tell where one should count 40 days from the moment of conception, or from the first day of the last menstruation, which is used in obstetrics. Only in the XX century has the connection between ovulation and fertilization been made.

Luckily from the thermodynamic viewpoint for man as a human biological system it is enough for him to consider, within him, solely the existence of a spiritual and material state, as co-existing entities. In that way, they must exist from the beginning of his existence that is from the moment of conception" [1]. Summarizing this review I generalize these considerations with the following points:

1. In the world's most famous equation of A. Einstein E=mc^2 the coefficient of time (the speed of light squared) does not change the identity of mass and energy, and each necessity of defining these concepts defining reality results from not taking into consideration information, which in inextricably bound with them in this equation.
2. The formula of transformation of reality E $\underline{\leftarrow i \rightarrow}$ mc^2 takes into consideration information both in the system and in the environment as co-existing and interacting together with both mass and energy.
3. The beginning of human life on the informational level of coexistence of spontaneous changes in the mass and energy of elementary particles requires, in social life, the acceptance of natural laws above those of man, because for the preservation of the species Homo Sapiens even the free will of humans is subject to the laws of thermodynamics.
4. Faith is the oldest source of knowledge about reality consisting of mass, information, and energy, the interaction of which is described by the formula E $\underline{\leftarrow i \rightarrow}$ mc^2 , pertaining to the common spontaneous exchange of mass and energy of elementary particles, including the information about their state and their environment.

Conflict of interest: I confirm that this review content has no conflict of interest.

Disclosure: This review article is an update of previously published articles entitled: "Causal prevention of cancer as a natural biological phenomenon" [*Medicine Biology Environment*. 1989;18(2):8-10], "The use in obstetrics of quantum theory as well as modern technology to decrease the morbidity and mortality of newborns and mothers during iatrogenic induced delivery" [*Neuroendocrinology Letters* 2001; 22:5-8] and "Cesarean biography of cancers" [In: Humenik, I., Szaniszlo, I. A., Zolacova, Z., Eds. *Reproducne zdravie zeny w centre zajmu*. Bratislava: Wolters Kluger 2014, pp. 207-21].

References

[1] Klimek, R. Termodynamiczne rozważania nad początkiem duchowego życia człowieka. [Thermodynamics beginning of the spiritual life of man]. *Gin. Pol.* 1990; 61(2): 90-97.

[2] Fedor-Freybergh, P. G., Maas, L. Continuity and indivisibility of integrated psychological, spiritual and somatic life processes. *Int. J. Prenat. Perinat. Psychol. Medicine* 2011; 23, suppl. 1, pp. 135-42.

[3] Jan Paweł, I. I. *Mądrość*. [Wisdom]. Kraków: UPJPII 2013.

[4] Klimek, R. Cell as a biological form of life. *Ginekol. i Położn.* 2007; 3 (5): 9-17.

[5] Khroutski, K. S. Forming an evolutionary vector to the Aristotelian Pole of scientific Organicism. *Biocosmology-neoAristotelism* 2013; Vol. 3(1) pp. 28-52. URL://en.biocosmology.ru/electronic-journal-biocosmology---neo-aristotelism.

[6] Klimek, R. Dekalog jako teologiczny program Świętej Trójcy w stworzeniu świata. [Ten Commandments-Holy Trinity teleological program of universe creation]. In: Jamrozy, M., Kuźmicz, A., Wszołek, B., Eds. *Człowiek i Wszechświat*. [Man and the Universe]. Częstochowa: 2012; 59-68.

[7] Kurjak, A., Chervenak, F. A., Eds. *Controversies on the beginning of human life*. New Delhi: Jitendar 2008.

[8] Hodorowicz, S., Jasiczek, D., Klimek, R., Tadeusiewicz, R., Eds. *Rak i niepłodność. Prawda i mity medycyny*. [Cancer and infertility. Truth and myth of medicine]. Kraków-Warszawa: Trio 2011.

[9] Klimek, R., Kolenda, Z. Carcinogenic entropy. *Curr. Gynecol. Oncol.* 2013; 11(1): 10-20.

[10] Klimek, R., Jasiczek, D., Stencl, J., Eds. *Explained cause of cancer*. Polish Academy of Science: Cracow 2013.

[11] Klimek, R. Conquering cancer ourselves. *New trends in gynecology and obstetrics*. J. Libbey CIC s.r.l., Roma 1990; Vol. VI No 2: 53-117.

[12] *The Bible*. Poznań-Warszawa: Pallotinum 1994.

[13] zur Hausen, H. Intracellular surveillance of persisting viral infections. Human genital cancer results from deficient cellular control of pappilomavirus gene expression. *Lancet* 1986; 2(8505): 489-91.

[14] zur Hausen, H. Papillomaviruses and cancer: from basic studies to clinical application. *Nat. Rev. Cancer* 2002; 2(5): 342-50.

[15] zur Hausen, H. Pappillomaviruses in anogenital cancer as a model to understand the role of viruses in human cancers. *Cancer Res.* 1989; 49 (17): 4677-81.

[16] Klimek, M., Klimek, R., Mazanek-Mościcka, M. Preterm birth as an indicator of cancer risk for the mother. *It. J. Gynacol. Obstet.* 2002; 3: 73-77.

[17] Jasiczek, D., Kaim, I., Czajkowski, K. Historic discovery of natural thermodynamic cause of cancer. *Neurocrinol. Letters* 2012; 33(4): 101-11.

[18] Jasiczek, D., Klimek, R., Štencl, J., Tadeusiewicz, R., Tholt, M. Obstetrical prevention of human cancers. *Neuroencrinology Letters* 2012; 33(2): 118-23.

[19] Klimek, R. Profilaktyczno-terapeutyczne szczepienie przeciwko stanom przedrakowym szyjki macicy. [Prophylactic and therapeutic vaccination against precancerous states of uterine cervix]. *Gin. Prakt.* 2007; 15(2): 36-40.

[20] Klimek, R., Czajkowski, K., Kojs, Z., Szymański, W., Śpiewankiewicz, B. Psychoneurocybernetyczna etiopatogeneza raków. Psychoneuro-cybernetic etiopathogenesis of cancers. *Curr. Gynecol. Oncol.* 2013; 11(3):202-09.

[21] Wojtyła, K. *Osoba i czyn.* [Person and Deed]. Lublin: TN KUL 2000.

[22] Rudnicki, K. *The cosmological principles.* Kraków: UJ 1995.

[23] Hodorowicz, S., Klimek, R., Korohoda, W., Tadeusiewicz, R. Informacja i samoorganizacja jako pojęcia termodynamicznej medycyny. [Information and self-organization in thermodynamic medicine]. *Alma Mater* 2009; 110-111: 87-90.

[24] Tadeusiewicz, R. New Trends in Neurocybernetics. *Computer Methods in Materials Science.* 2010; 10(1): 1-7.

[25] Tadeusiewicz, R. Place and Role of Intelligent Systems in Computer Science. *Computer Methods in Materials Science* 2010; Vol. 10, No. 4, pp. 193-206.

[26] Wszołek, B., Koźmicz, A., Jamrozy, M., Eds. *Człowiek i Wszechświat. Man and the Universe.* Częstochowa: WSP 2012.

[27] Collins, F. S. The language of God. *A Scientist presents evidence for belief.* Free Press New York-London-Sydney 2006.

[28] Schenker, J. G. *Ethical dileman in perinatal medicine.* Jaypee Brothers Medical Pub. New Delhi 2010.

In: Psychoneurocybernetic Conquest ...
Editor: Rudolf Klimek
ISBN: 978-1-63483-272-4

Chapter 2

Gynecological Prevention of Iatrogenic Carcinogenesis

Rudolf Klimek[1,*] ***and Joseph G. Schenker***[2]
[1]Fertility Centre Cracow, Cracow, Poland
[2]Hebrew University, Hadassah Medical Center, Jerusalem, Israel

"In the modern way of living stress and human reproduction have a great impact on our life and function"

(J. G. Schenker 1992)

Abstract

Physicians should be well aware of the fact that every single action of the human organism leaves a mark meant to be an event main-full in time, which itself only exists in the event, not beside it or outside of it. Also, tissue is not only a collection of cells and relations between them, but exists within the boundaries of an organism as a whole, e.g., mother's organism decides about the life or the death of each fetal microsystem which develops as fast as the organism of the mother is far from its own natural homeostasis. Premature birth indicates that the mother has enough strength to start the pregnancy structurally and functionally, but not

* Corresponding author: Prof. Rudolf Klimek, Fertility Centre Cracow, Pl. Szczepanski 3, 31-011 Cracow, Poland. E-mail: mmklimek@cyfronet.pl, phone: +48601547436, fax: +48-12 4225684.

enough to bring the fetus to its full maturity. Consequently preterm delivery prevention not only contributes to the health of the fetus, but also to the life and health of the mother, especially with respect to neoplasm risks. Modern obstetrics has explained the relation of preterm births to cervical cancer which can be promoted among others by many gynecological factors as faulty prediction of birth date, instrumental labor as well as hypothalamic conditioned abortion and delivery of premature newborns. Thus, the assessment of the newborn's maturity is very important not only for child, but also for the mother as the index of the higher cancer risk.

Keywords: Cellular dissipatogenesis, cervical cancer, gynecological guidelines, iatrogenic carcinogenesis, immunopotentialization, Naegel's rule, newborns maturity, quantum

INTRODUCTION

Every person, fulfilling himself in social life with other people, is created through the unification of reproductive cells of his/her parents as a unique single cell (zygote) to uphold the species. Each zygote defines the unique identity of each person whose whole life is determined by free will and neoplasms with their own differentially unique identities. Mother's organism decides about the life or the death of each fetal microsystem which develops as fast as the organism of the mother is far from its own natural equilibrium. Premature birth indicates that the mother has enough strength to start the pregnancy structurally and functionally, but not enough to bring the fetus to its full maturity. Consequently preterm delivery prevention not only contributes to the health of the fetus, but also to the life and health of the mother, especially with respect to neoplasm risks. Oppositely, the development of the first neoplastic cell only extends the cellular form of life without the possibility of autonomous existence. Unfortunately, carcinogenesis cannot be eliminated, but illnesses which are caused by neoplastic cells can and should be treated, as they can be healed more often by directly fighting the pathogenic factors and indirectly strengthening the whole organism through neurohormonal therapy or immunopotentialisation with vaccines. Preterm birth is a major cause of neonatal mortality, responsible for 28% of neonatal deaths overall. Prosperously, the administration of antenatal corticosteroids to women at high risk of preterm birth is a powerful perinatal intervention to reduce neonatal mortality.

The effect of antenatal steroids to reduce mortality and morbidity among preterm infants in hospital settings in many countries is well established [1-3].

Modern obstetrics has explained the relation of preterm births to cervical cancer which can be promoted among others by many gynecological factors, like faulty prediction of birth date, instrumental labor as well as hypothalamic conditioned abortion and delivery of premature newborns, which occur in 50% of cases after 37th gestational week [4-6]. Thus, the direct assessment of the newborn's maturity is very important not only for child, but also for the mother as the index of the higher cancer risk. One of the most important contributions to perinatology was the development of a new score for postnatal clinical assessment of fetal maturity in newborn infants [7]. The clinical methods used to date do require the evaluation of 12 - 34 parameters, their point range is complex and their results are given on the scale of 10-50 points. New method of fetal maturity assessment offers a possibility of objective evaluation of maturity immediately after birth and do not take into account weight and fetal age, but refer directly to fetal maturity. The new scale is simple and produces comparable results encompassing full maturity in the range of only 6-12 points, while immature newborns have less than 6 points. Its publication encouraged the obstetricians performing birth-date prediction, which is nowadays possible with an accuracy of several days instead of weeks in order to prevent iatrogenic prematurity caused by unnecessary induction or labor because of so-called post-dates. The necessity is needed for reformulation of the published ultra-sonomatric standards, so as to render them clinically useful in regard of the fetuses of various gestational maturation rate [8-10]. Potential and causal conditions for preterm births fall within a wide range of factors, from genetic hereditary states to psycho-emotional procreative reactions. It should be also emphasised that the same factors are in a causal link with the occurrence of cervical cancer. The most dangerous and common, but at the same time the easiest to eliminate factors leading to them are the constantly increasing cases of abnormal course of pregnancy and birth due to iatrogenic and medial causes as well as long-term and inadequate use of contraceptive pills [11-13].

Quantized Fetal Maturation

Quantum mechanics and theory of relativity are the most important scientific achievements of the twentieth century, but in spite of the great technological progress in the production of medical instruments and means of communication, they have not been used to the full in medical procedures. Individual pregnancy ends with reaching full fetal maturity, which is neither mass nor time and cannot be assessed in grams or units of time. At the atomic level each subsequent new indivisible unit (quantum) of fetal maturity appears at a particular time which is inseparable from maturing fetal structures. Thus, accordingly to the quickness of appearance of the consecutive quanta some fetuses are already mature at $37^{0/7}$ postmenstrual week of gestation while the other ones have to mature until $43^{2/7}$. Technical quantization differs from physical one by the fact the scale of examined parameters is set on macro level in such a way as to make them multiples of a selected measure (technical quantum). The fetal maturity level can be evaluated immediately after labor through obligatory assessment of just six of the many possible newborn features: position of the limbs, elbow angle, its mobility, breast nipple, plantar creases and lanugo. For each of those features one can allocate from 0 to 2 points, which maximally gives 12 technical points (quanta) of full maturity [7]. The new index differs from generally known methods in the smaller range of allocated 9±1.5 points, and what is more important - the possibility of making the assessment during routine examination of newborn baby immediately after its birth [1, 8, 10, 15].

The new medical goal is the defense of humanity against those workers of the medical profession whose patients become the victims of their improper actions or only ideas (words), which can be illustrated by the clinical meaning of Naegele's rule, which based only on the date of last menstruation before the pregnancy enables us to determine expected delivery date with an accuracy of ±3 weeks [8, 9, 14, 18].

Meanwhile many people still cannot seem to understand the concept of an average value of any set, which features half the population on each side, for example the newly born infants. The norm of any occurrence has been accepted to be 95% of all observable events, which in reference to natural human birth encompasses three weeks before and after the middle day of the six-week interval during which the birth is expected to take place. This is why the expected date of the end of the physiological pregnancy should be determined with an accuracy of three days, not weeks. What more, many obstetricians still continue to assess fetal maturity according to fetal weight or calendar duration of pregnancy and on that premise they act too often improperly. Labor occurred at an improper time is a common obstetrical error, which finds confirmation among others in higher perinatal mortality indexes both at the beginning (weeks $37^{th}/38^{th}$) and the end (weeks $41^{st}/42^{nd}$) of birth occurrence range in humans.

The former is characterized by neglect of assistance in actual preterm labor one week before true individual term, and the latter by preterm labor induction or – even worse – attempts to bring belated assistance in post-mature fetuses, whose birth time has passed in the former weeks of the calendar scale of pregnancy duration.

Intergenerational Cellular Transmission of Life

The reproductive cells of the grandparents influence the unique identity of the parents, whose gametes in turn influence the cellular genome of their children. In this, gynecology has a special place by protecting the patients' health from their conception in accordance to the contemporary level of knowledge, avoiding iatrogenic mistakes. Therefore a single zygote, whose environment is also important for its future development, defines the unique identity of each person, whose life is determined by free will and neoplasms [16-20]. Every living cell, in order to function, must uphold its own metabolism through the exchange of matter, information, and energy with surrounding cells, as well as complementing their functions by producing hormones, enzymes, or antibodies to uphold the function of individual organs and the whole body. If for some reason this exchange becomes limited, the cell initially limits additional activity. Finally, in order to counter the demise of its cellular existence, the cell must change the cellular genome which controls the metabolism [6, 21-23]. Neoplasm extends the cell form of life by improving and minimizing its own metabolism and this takes place due to increase of dissipation of matter, information and energy in the environment. Neoplasm is one-time alive form. This fact results from their statistically conditioned self-organization in a unique biological organism, and they are only able to develop in that organism. Owing to such dissipation, a neoplasm reduces in life span of the organism, thereby reducing its own.

The unique genome of the original cancer cell and the clones as its subsequent cells is recognized as such and attacked by biophysical, biochemical, and by immunological mechanisms, which requires not only time, but a production of specific antibodies for each individual neoplasm. For example an immunotherapy using lactic acid bacteria differentiates itself from other therapies by the fact that the vaccine uses symbiotic cells (Lactobim), for which the human organism is a natural habitat [25]. This means the person does not mark his antigens as alien to his or her body, as would be the case in vaccines against pathogens.

This limits the possibility of post vaccine complications when using Lactobim. Also, an age-long symbiosis of man and symbiotic or saprophytic microorganisms has led to the evolution of many different of their strains, whose set differs depending on the environment of peoples' lives. Hence not only the type of symbiotic bacteria, but also the proportions of different strains have an influence on the efficacy of different vaccines, which take into account the physiological flora in the urogenital and gastrointestinal tracts maintaining the proper acidic base in these organs.

It is not only important to the organic functions themselves, but especially to the effectiveness of the immune system [2, 6]. The above facts may easily be connected with the huge impact of psycho-emotional attitudes of both physicians and patients, e.g., those iatrogenic treating mild acne symptoms with contraceptive pills, advertised as a new recommendation to improve facial beauty. After the periods of neonatal and fetal psycho-perinatology, medicine has reached the level of an individual human cell. About 20% of women with post-pregnancy neurohormonal insufficiency (hypothalamosis) have clinically recognised pre-cancer states of cervix, due to e.g., the history of obstetrical haemorrhages, abortions and pre-term births.

The production of hormones depends on the activity of its component enzymes, mainly on the clinical condition of endocrine glands, where biophysical processes are of great importance, since they are related both to atomic level of metabolism and purely physical blood flow and concentration of its components.

Therefore, as early as in the period of pregnancy fetal reproductive cells should be protected by taking care of gonads, due to their prime importance in the intergenerational passage of life and endocrine regulation of whole organism [5, 25, 26].

Cancer and Procreation

Procreation disorders lead mainly to neoplasms of reproductive organs, as improper diet favours neoplasms of the alimentary tract. Definitely, cervical cancer is not an infectious disease, but it must be remembered that infection, inflammation and infectious diseases weaken the biochemical, neurohormonal and immunological regulation of the organism, which makes it difficult to eliminated dissipathogenic states in every cellular metabolism [6, 21, 22]. According to medical thermodynamics, each infection may extremely depart cell from the physiological internal states.

Killing bacilli and preventing infection may symptomatically restrict or eliminate numerous infectious diseases, but to fight neoplasms as natural phenomena one must employ a completely new strategy, which may be compared to the strategy used in lightning rods or stations of early detection of potentially dangerous natural forces. Methods and measures used to achieve this goal must be implemented and advertised according to the current state of knowledge about them. Therefore, it is important not to neglect treatment of even the least advanced pre-cancer states, such as cervical intraepithelial neoplasia (CIN1) only because 50% of them disappear, since the other half leads to development of a neoplastic disease [14, 17, 21].

The clinical possibility of visualizing the dissipathogenic state of cells allows for an early identification of the localization and reach of pre-cancerous cells, which till now could be identified via cytology or histopathology. Such a dissipathogenic state, can be caused by many factors such as alcoholism, smoking, malnutrition, excessive physical exertion, infections, and the ageing of the body.

It can be affected in: the digestive tract (type of food, its preparation and storage), the circulatory and pulmonary system (environmental damage), neurohormonal system (stress, hormone therapy, infertility), the reproductive system in women (number and type of pregnancies and miscarriages, uterine bleeding, lack of lactation). Finally, a direct effect on the cells of not only stable (tissue) and unstable human ones (white and red blood cells, microphages, lymphocytes, etcetera), but also saprophytic and pathogenic single cellular organisms, which, apart from competing for their own existence also act in defense against germs.

The conventional treatment of neoplastic illnesses is based on combating each of the aforementioned factors and/or many of them together.

As soon as a patient is diagnosed with a neoplastic illness, it is necessary not only to remove the neoplasm from the organism, but to also return the cells surrounding it to their original states of internal balance, especially if they are already in a dissipathogenic state.

In social life truth, love and responsibility are some of the most fundamental properties of reliable information. Unfortunately, for diverse personal reasons, information is often used to agitate for harmful ideas. This happens despite introduction of neuroendocrinological and immunological therapy of even preneoplastic states, the nucleomagnetic resonance diagnosis of those states and modern thermodynamic treatment of all neoplasms; and it happens even though it has been proven that gynaecologists contribute to the increased incidence of the best understood cancer, that is cervical cancer.

Apart from the dissipative self-organization of cellular forms of life neoplasm also applies to a person's psychological and social life in the form of long known psychoses and newly described informative disease (informatonosis).

Conclusion

In the twentieth century medicine was linked with psychology by the examination of psychological states on the atomic level due to the introduction of spectroscopy of the inside of the organism's cells via nuclear magnetic resonance, which can help to determine e.g., the potential places of neoplastic self-organization or even speech disruptions depending on the gender of the patient. This helped to introduce the photodynamic treatment of neoplasm, saving healthy tissue without the need for surgical interference. The uniqueness of each neoplastic disease is based on the fact that humans need their treatment to be accompanied by therapy and rehabilitation of the primary illness while taking into consideration the ageing process itself.

Only the psycho-emotional state of a person does not have an end to its existence as opposed to the cellular forms of life and their possible neoplastic end form. This includes gametes as well, with the exception of those which were statistically chosen to create new zygotes in the process of continuation of the next unique, purely informational human existence. This not only explains the emergence of neoplasm already in the fetus, but also the lack of other oncological hazards in the life of the oncologically ill due to their family history of this illness.

For many years neogenesis was seen in terms of the role of oncogenes, until the proponents of this theory convinced themselves that the unit of hereditary traits consists not only of nuclear DNA, which can be used sole to select the type and efficacy of treatment. The same goes for the infectious etiology of neoplasm, advertised by individuals believing only in their own ideas, despite tried and tested medical rules. The twenty-first century started with the domination of information, which turns the focus upon the meaning of the moral-ethic dimension of humanity. Therefore, the modern gynecologic rules in relation to psycho-oncology must accept following prohibitions concerning: 1. Using a cesarean section solely based upon the wish of the mother as an expression of the lack of sufficient psycho-prophylactic of birth; 2. Inducing the birth solely based upon the duration of the pregnancy, especially when accompanied by obstetric diabetes; 3. A reduction of the number of embryos in pregnancies following an assisted treatment of infertility; 4. Treating infertility without taking the health state of both parents into account; 5. Using hormonal systems of contraception for any other reason than prevention of pregnancy, which does not preclude using the hormones in diagnostics and endocrinological therapy. Also the most important gynecological guidelines used for the last 15 years should be changed at least into the following imperatives: 1. Specify the actual date of the birth with an accuracy of ± 3 days with the use of obstetric imaging (USG, MRI) instead of making only a probable estimate using Naegele's rule with the accuracy of ± three weeks; 2. Specify the sensitivity of the contractions of the uterus when determining the date of birth, compulsory before birth induction; 3 Enzymatic monitor the development of the pregnancy and make prognoses as to the birth process, determining maternal blood oxytocinases; 4. Use the ACTH-depot therapy instead of betametazone and dexametazone; 5. Compulsory determination of the new born maturity level instead of solely his/her pulmonary adaptation immediately after each delivery.

Conflict of interest: The authors confirm that this article content has no conflict of interest.

References

[1] Hodorowicz, S., Jasiczek, D., Klimek, R., Tadeusiewicz, R., Eds. *Rak i niepłodność. Prawda i mity medycyny.* [Cancer and infertility. Truth and myth of medicine]. Kraków-Warszawa Trio 2011.

[2] Schenker, J. G. Stress and human reproduction. In: Klimek, R., Ed. *Pre-Peri-Natal Psycho-Medicine* 1992; DreAM Cracow, p. 77-82.

[3] Schenker, J. G. *Ethical dilemas in perinatal medicine.* New Delhi: Jaypee Brothers Medical Pub. 2010.

[4] Jasiczek, D., Kaim, I., Czajkowski, K. Historic discovery of natural thermodynamic cause of cancer. *Neurocrinol. Lett.* 2012; 33(4): 101-111.

[5] Klimek, M., Klimek, R., Mazanek-Mościcka, M. Preterm birth as an indicator of cancer risk for the mother. *It. J. Gynacol. Obstet.* 2002; 3: 73-77.

[6] Klimek, R., Jasiczek, D., Stencl, J. *Explained cause of cancer.* Polish Academy of Science 2013; Cracow.

[7] Klimek, R., Klimek, M., Rzepecka-Weglarz, B. A new score for postnatal clinical assessment of fetal maturity in newborn infants. *Int. J. Obstet. Gynecol.* 2000; 71: 101-105.

[8] Cosmi, E. V., Klimek, R., Di Renzo, G. C., et al. Prognosis of birth term: recommendations on current practice and overview of new developments. *Archives of Perinatal Medicine* 1997; 3(2): 31-50.

[9] Klimek, R. *Monitoring of pregnancy and prediction of birth date.* The Parthenon Publishing Group 1994; New York, London.

[10] Klimek, R., Bręborowicz, G. H., Chazan, B., et al. Declaration of the Childbirth in XXI century. *Archives of Perinatal Medicine* 2001; 7(3), 8-14.

[11] De Marco, F., Bucaj, E., Foppoli, C., et al. Oxidative stress in HPV-Driven Viral Carcinogenesis: Redox Proteomics Analysis of HPV-16 Dysplastic and Neoplastic Tissues. *PLoS One* 2012; 7(13): e34366.

[12] Fedor-Freybergh, P. G., Maas, L. Continuity and indivisibility of integrated psychological, spiritual and somatic life processes. *Int. J. Prenat. Perinat. Psychol. Medicine* 2011; 23, Suppl. 1, pp. 135-42.

[13] Klimek, R., Klimek, M., Gralek, P., Jasiczek, D. Causal ACTH-depot therapy during pregnancies following infertility treatment. *Obstetrics Gynecology International 2012*; Volume 2012, article ID 248926, 7 p.

[14] Jasiczek, D., Klimek, R., Štencl, J., Tadeusiewicz, R., Tholt, M. Obstetrical prevention of human cancers. *Neuroencrinology Letters* 2012;33(2): 118-23.

[15] Klimek, M., Klimek, R., Skotniczny, K., et al. Auxiological relations between prenatal ultrasound and oxitocinase measurements high-risk pregnancies. *J. Prenat. Neonat. Med.* 2001; 6: 350-55.

[16] Klimek, R. Cell as a biological form of life. *Ginekol i Położn* 2007; 3(5): 9-17.

[17] Klimek, R., Jasiczek, D., Gralek, P., Fedor-Freybergh, P. Cancer – final cellular form of life. *Int. J. Prenat. Psychol. Medicine* 2011; 23: 1-2: 7-17.

[18] Kurjak, A., Chervenak, F. A., Eds. *Controversies on the beginning of human life.* Jitendar 2008; New Delhi.

[19] Schiffman, M., Wentzensen, N. From human papillomavirus to cervical cancer. *Obstetrics and Gynecology* 2010; 116(1): 177-85.

[20] Tadeusiewicz, R. Place and Role of Intelligent Systems in Computer Science. *Computer Methods in Materials Science* 2010; Vol. 10, No. 4, pp. 193-206.

[21] Klimek, R. NMR imaginig in terms of human atomic patology. *Europ. J. Obstet. Gyn. and Reproductive Biology* 1987; 24(2): 135-43.
[22] Klimek, R. Nuclear magnetic resonance in obstetrics and gynecology. *Int. J. Gynecol. Obstet.* 1990; 32: 199-205.
[23] Klimek, R., Kolenda, Z. Carcinogenic entropy. *Curr. Gynecol. Oncol.* 2013; 11(1): 10-20.
[24] Kolenda, Z., et al. On the Minimum Entropy Production in Steady-State Heat Conduction Processes. *Energy*, Elsevier 2004; vol. 29 pp. 2441-60.
[25] Klimek, R., Klimek, M., Jasiczek, D. Immunotherapy of cervical cancer as a biological dissipative structure. *Neuroendocrinology Letters* 2011; 32(4): 380-88.
[26] Klimek, M. The Effectiveness of Adrenocorticotropin Repeated Doses in High Risk Pregnancies. *Fetal Diagn. Ther.* 2006; 21: 528-31.

In: Psychoneurocybernetic Conquest ... ISBN: 978-1-63483-272-4
Editor: Rudolf Klimek

Chapter 3

OBSTETRICAL INFORMATONOSIS - DIAGNOSIS AND TREATMENT

***Krzysztof Czajkowski*[1], *Rudolf Klimek*[2,*], *Lubomira Panikova*[3], *Jerzy Sikora*[4], *Jan Stencl*[5], *Marian Tholt*[3], *Michal Valent*[5] *and Pavel Ventruba*[6]**

[1]Warsaw Medical University, Warsaw, Poland
[2]Fertility Centre Cracow, Poland
[3]Hospital Trstena, Slovakia
[4]Silesia Medical University Katowice, Poland
[5]Slovak Medical University Bratislava, Slovakia
[6]Masaryk University Brno, Czech Republic

ABSTRACT

Humans view their own consciousness as the non-material motivation for their lives and actions according to their own values of social life. The social form of people's lives is emphasized by information expressed by words, where the word has actuating power. Although a lot of information is passed on as true and correct, their source is not always known, or who has created it for what reason, or in what surroundings it manifests itself. Often, the information is inaccurate, superfluous, or pertains only to a very narrow group of illnesses, yet is treated as a

* Corresponding author: Prof. Rudolf Klimek, Fertility Centre Cracow, Poland. E-mail: mmklimek@cyfronet.pl, phone: +48601547436, fax: +48-12 4225684.

universal communication. 'Informatonosis' is the name given to an illness which is detrimental to personal as well as social health, and the cause of which is information generated by humans. The effects of any given information are not always directly foreseeable. We have a deep belief that, except under unusual circumstances, information is spread in good faith, due to a need for action or the necessity to identify and obtain relatively simple rules of conduct. Unfortunately, sometimes the information is based upon seemingly correct theoretical assumptions, ones still not proven in clinical practice, or pertains to too small or too specific groups of patients, but is spread as if it was a tried and tested diagnostic method or therapy. In such a way, not only medical advances are popularized (whether by design or not), but also an induction of informatonosis occurs. In the history of medicine, many examples can be found where an accepted form of therapy or diagnosis, after many years, has not yielded the expected efficacy. Only years of research, additionally confronted with a recent state of knowledge (not only medical) possess current value.

Keywords: Apgar score, high-risk pregnancy, carcinogenesis, informatonosis, obstetrical prevention, diagnosis and therapy, preterm deliveries, newborns maturity index

INTRODUCTION

Obstetrics and gynecology, like every medical specialization, use human knowledge and the skill of its practical application in order to treat, protect and heal, as well as rehabilitate. Obstetrics is, however, a special field of medicine. It is concerned with a person's health from conception to their material-energetic demise. In opposition to other medical fields obstetrics is often concerned with healthy individuals, not only in the obstetric aspect, but in all procreation, including the prevention of illness, and even (in concurrence with current law) sometimes unfortunately with the elimination of individuals considered ill. In many situations, the possibility of the observation of a developing child is limited, and a 100% correct confirmation of the observations is impossible before the pregnancy is over. Often, the undertaken diagnostic and therapeutic actions are more the result of a need for action than of existing scientific facts [1-6]. The essence of life is a spontaneous, constant and common exchange of matter and energy of elementary particles, including information about their state, a phenomenon observed on the atomic level, on which single and multicellular organisms exist, until shortly believed to be the only living structures [3, 7-10]. Humans observe the surrounding reality with their senses and try to define their consciousness (their "I") as a non-material motivation for their life and actions according to their own values of social life. The social form of people's lives is emphasized by information expressed by words, where the word has actuating power, although it can be interpreted in various ways. Equally important is their source, or who has created it for what reason, or in what surrounding it manifests itself. It is on this that a new type of illness is based, the cause of which is information generated by humans (usually not aware of its distant effects) which is detrimental to personal as well as social health. It was named 'informatonosis' to differentiate it from zoonosis, which are illnesses of animal origin. The uniqueness of this illness is a result of a purely informational base of detrimental actions and behavior of such people, called 'informatonotics [11-13].

In this article, we discuss the recent advances in the discovery of cancers as self-organized dissipative biological structures, their relevance for early gynecological prevention, detection and causal therapy, particularly in women during pregnancy.

Diagnosis of Illnesses Caused by Medical Information

The medical inseparability of theory and practice aids in the diagnosis of informatonosis in ill doctors. It manifests itself in views and actions detrimental to the health of patients, resulting from negative personal or acquired beliefs in social life. An example of informatonosis would be an obstetrician who publicly protests against a damaging increase in the frequency of operative births via cesarean section, and yet is ready to use a cesarean section in his own obstetrical unit without any medical indications. On the other hand, a form of informatonosis would be a tolerance of crossing the 15% threshold of performed cesarean sections. Despite the only fully physiological form of birth being a natural one, there is a constant move toward increasing the indications for a cesarean section, in order to minimalize possible complications for mother and child in a natural birth. From a statistical point of view a higher or lower percentage of cesarean sections is a subject for more or less scientific contemplations. From the point of view of the family, raising a child damaged during the birth process – a cesarean section is a chance for a healthy child.

An alarmingly high percentage of cesarean sections would indicate an informatonosis of the individuals responsible for this. On one hand one may, for the patient, paint a picture of complications during birth (which don't always exist), and on the other hand, an exact date of the birth, predicable to the hour would be very suitable for both the doctor and the mother, for whom the pregnancy and birth are only dates in a calendar (but let us hope important ones). In this aspect using medical knowledge to determine 'medical indications' for a cesarean section would be a form of informatonosis, unless we officially include the mother's wish for a cesarean section in the group of medical indicators [1, 5, 14].

An illness caused by information can apply to a single person, authors of incorrect manuals, as well as the creators of incorrectly programmed medical tools. For example, the expected date of delivery (EDD) is one of the most commonly found units of information connected with both the prognosis of a birth and an ex post assessment of it, especially of one performed operatively. It is known that according to the date of the last menstruation period the date of birth can be statistically determined with a precision of plus/minus three weeks. Performing an ultrasonography is very helpful in such a case as it helps to determine various aspects of the foetus. After inserting the measurements into the computer it checks which 50 percentile of the week of pregnancy the size of the foetus corresponds to. The potential error of ± 7-10 days in the first 10 weeks of pregnancy, ± 2 weeks in its middle and ± 3 weeks at its end is a result of the mean dynamics of the foetal growth. Convincing oneself as well as the mother that the statistical date of birth can be determined extremely precisely and that this date is some sort of deadline is a form of informatonosis leading to many unnecessary inductions of birth after 40 weeks of pregnancy [15-18]. Unfortunately often one falsely assumes a limit of 37 weeks (259 days) of the pregnancy to determine premature births, thus missing a whole half (!) of all births of premature infants in the later stages, considering them to be 'newborn with a low birth mass' (?). In order to avoid taking responsibility for thus causing prematurity, the Apgar scale is used. This scale was originally developed by anesthesiologists to decide on the effect of anesthesia on the newborn and not solely the level of post-birth pulmonary adaptation. Of course a mature foetus has high marks on the Apgar scale. It is also known that in multiple-foetus pregnancies, in mothers with high blood pressure, obesity, diabetes and/or neurohormonal insufficiency, and even in a coexisting neoplastic illness, many foetuses are characterized by an accelerated intrauterine maturing process [5, 19-21].

A premature child can be determined independently from the duration of the pregnancy, the height and the body mass. More than half of all fetuses are still immature before the date calculated in accordance with Naegele's rules, and a week after that - every fifth fetus should still be maturing in the mother's womb. Therefore, pregnant women should be monitored using ultrasound for the speed of the fetal maturation rate to predict in which of the six weeks of the human birthing norm the birth is to take place. As a result, during this time the obstetricians do not provide the necessary assistance to pregnant women in the event of both premature birth and a pregnancy which moves beyond the determined real date of birth, but instead all too often initiate a birth a week or more before the foetus has matured. In addition, a cesarean section deprives the child of a natural adaptation in the mother's birth canal to help it begin an independent life. A cesarean section, regardless of the indication and stage of pregnancy is linked with a significantly higher risk of intermittent respiratory disruption in the child, especially if it is prevented from a pre-birth 3-4 day preparation of the heart for a sudden change in blood circulation. The maturation of the lungs of the foetus is also ended earlier, but it can luckily be strengthened by administering synthetic corticoids in case of an impending premature birth. Unfortunately this (very often a last resort) is a result of the lack of understanding the involvement of hypothalamo-hypophyseal-adrenal axis in perinatology [22, 23]. The actions of the doctors responsible for this can be justified only by their informational illness – informatonosis. In its early stage it is treatable due to effective social information, but already as a psychosis since medical responsibility can make it fall under legal jurisdiction. Another unwanted iatrogenic effect of a cesarean section performed before the due date can be, as results of studies show, a predisposition to endometric changes in the postoperative wound of the abdomen [24-26].

Causal Treatment of Informatonosis

Every event in nature is always a result of its own cause, the discovery of which has a major meaning in medicine. The biggest difficulty was the discovery of the thermodynamic reasons for the development of neoplasm in the ill person, which, as multicellular biological structure, have a unique genetic identity, which was until recently linked with large number of oncogenic factors. It is enough to understand that each cell of the organism exists due to the exchange of matter, energy and information with its cellular surroundings, and in a state of internal metabolic equilibrium it additionally produces hormones, enzymes, antibodies, etc. in order to support the whole organism. In the case of an extreme disruption of cellular metabolism it not only ceases external functions, but in order to prolong its own life it must undergo self-organization into a more efficient structure while increasing the dissipation of matter and energy in its surroundings [2-4]. This internal state, furthest from its own equilibrium, is called 'dissipathogenic', and is that long sought after cause of neoplasms. The cells in a dissipathogenic state still belong to clones of cells created from the zygote, but after the neoplastic transformation they form a unique cellular structure with a new genome, but are adapted to life only in their current surroundings. Due to the introduction of imaging and spectroscopy using magnetic resonance medicine has reached the atomic level of the organism [12, 24]. Unfortunately doctors are seldom aware of the universal laws of thermodynamics, the use of which has already changed terminology and medical technology. Some gynecologists, for example, instead of correcting their iatrogenic actions do not learn the basic principles (entropy, dissipation), and try to explain the etiopathogenesis of cervical cancer with a viral infection. Apart from the known intracellular disorders created by the penetration of the virus into the cell's genome, the cell's dissipathogenic state must arise resulting in the fact that neoplasm develops only in some women infected with the virus. The pathogenic microorganisms are the cause of infectious diseases, but the infection with them itself not always causes local afflictions and symptoms if the body's immune system is effective. If a treatment based on the destruction of the microorganisms is not possible, then an indirect strengthening of the immune forces together with strengthening saprophytic microorganisms can help fight dangerous (also for them) pathogens (viruses, chlamydia, pathogenic bacteria, etc.). Proving the cause-effect link is essential in order to differentiate the cause from factors deciding the cause's efficacy, because the same cause can have different effects. An inflammation of tissue, apart from infections, can be caused by thermic or radioactive radiation, or even by chemical agents, while infections in women are influenced by age, number of sexual patients, the time and type of contraceptives used, drug use, etc. Medicine must, on one hand, accept the role of whole body factors, and on the other – the results of genetic examinations pertaining to hereditary dangers like breast or ovarian cancer, or even diabetes. To avoid iatrogenic effects one must constantly remember that these are necessary but insufficient oncogenic factors.

The explanation of the cause of neoplastic illnesses creates an example for the treatment of informatonosis, because even solely its understanding can return a normal psycho-emotional state in these persons.

The treatment of informatonosis depends on the suggested in the hippocratic oath the necessity of self-education, and in extreme cases on compulsory constant education. But this is not enough in cases of the most advanced information psychoses, which show a dissipative psycho-emotional self-organization of the personality, manifesting a so-called "obstetric terrorism." The most effective treatment lies in demonstrating the results of those doctors who, in accordance with nature and their professional calling, achieve a low perinatal mortality (2.2‰) with 16% of cesarean sections of all births. The explanation of mistakes must be documented by way of prophylactics and patient treatment. This applies also to the criteria of epidemological analyses of their illnesses and mortality, and in the case of obstetrics – foetuses, infants and mothers. For example in the year 2012 in the hospital of Trsten in Slovak Tatras it was noted: 46 infants born as premature children according to the criterium of the length of the pregnancy before 37 weeks, in which 30 had a mass ≥ 2500g, therefore fulfilled the classical lower limit of foetal maturity and a whole 14 of them also had a body length ≥ 48 cm. This stays in accordance with the results of prospective examinations of over 56 thousand births in an adjacent part of Poland, in which the two mentioned criteria were fulfilled by only 2.5% of all infants [19, 12]. The main cause of increase in the percentage of cesarean sections should be considered an extension of obstetric and non-obstetric indications. During the 30 years' activities of Medical University of Toruń held 69366 births, of which 11814 by cesarean section (17.03%), covering the period 1980-2009 a steady increasing number of cesarean section performed from 9.35% to 28.13% and reduction in procedures using forceps from 1.5% to 0.63%, and a manual assistance from 3.5% to 0.63%. Indications for cesarean section because of the state of the treatment of infertility covered similar percentage of pregnant women, but statistically significantly reduced the number of indication due to maternal age. No one was performed according only to wish of mother [25].

Half of all recurring miscarriages still surprise obstetricians, who not only do not use enzymatic monitoring (with the help of oxytocinase) which has been known for fifty years, but also do not examine the essential hypothalamo-hypophyseal-adrenal axis [1, 21]. They use excessive gonadotropins, but do not underestimate the meaning of adrenocorticotrophin, or even block it with synthetic steroid drugs without determining the ACTH levels in the blood of the mother. Moreover, they justify the excessive number of induced and operative births by the accumulation of pathology in their obstetrics units, which they often cause themselves through their action or non-action, the best example of which is the endometriosis of abdominal epithel in scars after cesarean sections which were performed too early before the tolerance of the foetal tissues of the mother's organism ended [26].

Conclusion

The most commonly known historical incident involving deformities caused by producers of pharmaceuticals and medical equipment is the birth of children with deformed or missing extremities as an effect of ingesting only a few tablets of Talidomid during pregnancy, advertised as a safe drug against nausea. This serves to remind that in the last few days of the child's life inside the mother, many processes occur which are essential to the beginning and ending of the birth process. A lack of responsibility is demonstrated by setting the date of birth based solely on the date of the last period only because the patient is seen as a statistic, not a real entity. To neglect giving birth at the correct moment can be compared to the harmfulness of Talidomid in early pregnancy, with the difference being the cause of injury to the child is not from a specific drug with proven harmful effects. In both situations, a time frame of only a few days is involved. In the first case, one can prove the fact of administering or ingesting the harmful substance. In the second case, it is difficult to determine the individual responsibility, although the harmfulness of statistically, medically and demographically documented cesarean sections done without medical indications, iatrogenic premature births, and prematurity are not justified in a specific medical situation lies beyond doubt. They can be substantially lowered through the individualization of medical care, using common methods of increasing the precision of predicting the date of birth, or as simply and easily as the counting of Apgar points, and determining the level of foetal maturity of born children to document the correct choice of the date of birth in an objective way [1, 5, 16].

Conflict of interest: The authors confirm that this article content has no conflict of interest.

Disclosure: This review article is an update of previously published manuscripts entitled: Cell as a biological form of life [3], Information and self-organization in thermodynamic medicine [7], Informatonosis – an information disease affecting the society [11], Obstetrical prevention of human cancers [19].

REFERENCES

[1] Czajkowski, K., Szymański, Eds. *Rudolfa Klimka Położnictwo*. [R. Klimek's Obstetrics]. RK, Kraków 2006.
[2] Klimek, R. Cervical cancer as a natural phenomenon. *Eur. J. Obstet. Gynecol. Reprod. Biol.* 1990; 36: 221-238.
[3] Klimek, R. Cell as a biological form of life. *Ginekol. Położn.* 2007; 3: 9-17.
[4] Klimek, R. Cancer: health hazard resulting from attempted life protection. *Curr. Gynecol. Oncol.* 2010; 8: 149-159.
[5] Klimek, R., Bręborowicz, G. H., Chazan, B. Declaration of the Childbirth in XXI century. *Arch. Perinat. Med.* 2001; 7(3), 8-14.
[6] Klimek, R., Jasiczek, D., Gralek, P., Fedor-Freybergh, P. Cancer – final cellular form of life. *Int. J. Prenat. Perinat. Psychol. Medicine* 2011; 23: 7-17.
[7] Hodorowicz, S., Klimek, R., Korohoda, W., Tadeusiewicz, R. Informacja i samoorganizacja jako pojęcia termodynamicznej medycyny. [Information and self-organization in thermodynamic medicine]. *Alma Mater* 2009; 110-111: 87-90.
[8] Hodorowicz, S., Jasiczek, D., Klimek, R., Tadeusiewicz, R. *Rak i niepłodność. Prawda i mity medycyny*. [Cancer and infertility. Truth and myth of medicine]. Kraków – Warszawa: Trio 2011.
[9] Jasiczek, D., Kaim, I., Czajkowski, K. Historic discovery of natural thermodynamic cause of cancer. *Neuroendocrinol. Lett.* 2012; 33: 361-371.
[10] Mazanek-Mościcka, M., Pabian, W. The Cracow Obstetrical School – main achivements. *Arch. Perinat. Med.* 2001; 7(3):37-41.
[11] Jasiczek, D., Klimek, R. Informatonosis – an information disease affecting the society. *Int. J. Prenat. Perinat. Psychol. Medicine* 2013; 25: 22-31.
[12] Klimek, R., Jasiczek, D., Stencl, J., Eds. *Explained cause of cancer*. Cracow: Hermes Management 2013.
[13] Wszołek, B., Kuźmicz, A., Jamrozy, M. Eds. *Człowiek i Wszechświat*. The Man and the Univers. Częstochowa: WSP 2012.
[14] Cosmi, E. V., Klimek, R., Di Renzo, G. C., et al. Prognosis of birth term: recommendations on current practice and overview of new developments. *Arch. Perinat. Med.* 1997; 3(2): 31-50.

[15] Hajek, Z., Haakova, L., Kolarik, D., et al. Operative deliveries, professional and economic aspects. *Arch. Perinat. Med.* 2001; 7(3): 30-32.

[16] Klimek, M. Prediction of the birth term and course of the labor. *Arch. Perinat. Med.* 2001; 7(3): 24-29.

[17] Klimek, M., Klimek, R., Mazanek-Mościcka, M. Preterm birth as an indicator of cancer risk for the mother. *It. J. Gynaecol. Obstet.* 2002; 3: 73-77.

[18] Roztocil, A., Koudelka, M., Jelinek, J., et al. Elective induction of labour. A benefis to the mother and foetus/neonate or an obstetric hazard? *Int. J. Pre- and Perinatal Psych. Med.* 1997; 9(3): 299-306.

[19] Jasiczek, D., Klimek, R., Štencl, J., Tdeusiewicz, R., Thold, M. Obstetrical prevention of human cancers. *Neuroendocrinol. Lett.* 2012; 33: 118-123.

[20] Klimek, R., Klimek, M., Gralek, P., Jasiczek, D. Causal ACTH-depot therapy during pregnancies following infertility treatment. *Obstet. Gynecol. Int.* 2012; 248926.

[21] Klimek, R., Lauterbach, R. Posnatal clinical assessment of fetal maturity in new born infants. *Arch. Perinat. Med.* 2001; 7(3): 19-23.

[22] Gałązka, K., Pityński, K., Skręt-Magiełło, J., et al. The increase in metallothionein eutopic and ectipic decidual immunoreactivity with respect to the progression of labor term and lack of analogical changes in placental abruption. *Am. J. Reprod. Immunol.* 2008; 60: 204-213.

[23] Klimek, R., Klimek, M., Jasiczek, D. Immunotherapy of cervical cancer as a biological dissipative structure. *Neuroendocrinol. Lett.* 2011; 32: 380-388.

[24] Klimek, R., Madej, J. M., Sieroń, A. Eds. *Rak – nowotwory a choroby nowotworowe*. [Cancer – neoplasms and neoplastic diseases]. Kraków: RK 2006.

[25] Kolesińska-Konkel, N. *Analysis of indicacions for operative deliveries*. [MD thesis] Toruń-Bydgoszcz: UMK 2013.

[26] Skręt-Magiełło, J., Wicherek, L., Basta, P., et al. RCAS1 decidual immunoreactivity during the cesarean section scar. Deciduosis immune cell presence and activity. *Gin. Obst. Invest.* 2008; 65: 187-194.

In: Psychoneurocybernetic Conquest … ISBN: 978-1-63483-272-4
Editor: Rudolf Klimek

Chapter 4

NEOVASCULARIZATION AND NEOANGIOGENESIS IN DIFFERENTIATING ADNEXAL LESIONS WITH CONTRAST-ENHANCED TRANSVAGINAL ULTRASOUND

Marek Szymanski*
Department and Clinic of Obstetrics, Gynecology and Oncological Gynecology, Collegium Medicum, Nicolaus Copernicus University in Toruń, Poland

ABSTRACT

Objectives: To analyze the relationship between contrasting kinetics in the tumorous vessels and histological type of the lesion in attempt to differentiate between a malignant and benign disease.

Methods: One-hundred sixty patients were hospitalized due to diagnosis of unilateral or bilateral adnexal masses and referred to elective surgeons; they underwent contrast-enhanced ultrasound examination (CEUS). The contrast kinetics were obtained and compared with the neovascularization parameters of the studied lesions.

* Corresponding author: Marek Szymański, Department and Clinic of Obstetrics, Gynecology and Oncological Gynecology Collegium Medicum in Bydgoszcz, Ujejskiego 75 Str. 85-168 Bydgoszcz, Poland. Phone: +48 601 848 984, fax: +48 52 349 06 45, e-mail: szymar@hoga.pl.

Results: Fifty-one malignant and benign lesions comprised the final analysis. Diagnostic time-intensity curves were constructed for all patients. Baseline and maximum color Doppler intensities, as well as the absolute and relative increases in color Doppler intensity, were significantly higher ($p<0.0001$) in malignant tumors than they were in benign tumors. Peak enhanced intensity of fractional color Doppler Area (%CDA) and area under time-intensity curve (S-parameter) correlated significantly with the histological character of the lesion $p<0.0001$. The larger the value of the S-parameter, the higher the risk of malignant tumor character of the lesion.

Conclusion: The accuracy of contrast-enhanced transvaginal ultrasound was higher than grey scale assessment at differentiating between benign and malignant adnexal lesions.

Keywords: Contrast enhanced ultrasound, neovascularization, neoangiogenesis, ovarian cancer

ABBREVIATIONS

US	ultrasound
FIGO	The International Federation of Gynecologists and Obstetricians
CEUS	contrast-enhanced ultrasound
IOTA	International Ovarian Tumor Analysis
CQ	color quantifier (software)
ROI	region of interest
%CDA	fractional Color Doppler area
AUC	area under curve
SD	standard deviation
OR	odds ratio
CI	confidence intervals

INTRODUCTION

Transvaginal ultrasound (US) examination still represents the most convenient method for evaluation of pelvic masses and in particular early diagnosis of adnexal lesions [1]. Its use is advocated by current international guidelines as the modality of first choice in patients with a suspicious isolated ovarian mass [2]. Owing to certain limitations, like the lack of reflection from red blood cells and low signal to noise ratio, conventional power Doppler, however, displays limited sensitivity (50-80%) and specificity (80-90%), [3-5] for distinguishing benign tumors from malignant tumors.

Because of commonly delayed diagnoses, ovarian cancer is associated with poor prognosis, with a 5-year survival rates ranging from 27% to 16% respectively for FIGO-stage III and IV. For those patients, all recent advancement implementations, including radical surgery and new chemotherapy treatment modalities, result only in a prolongation of survival, but not in a significant improvement of the cure rate after 6–8 years [6, 7]. Therefore, early detection and proper diagnosis of an early-stage disease is of great importance with presumed impact on the prognosis.

Several observational studies have investigated the role of contrast-enhanced US (CEUS) in the diagnosis of ovarian tumors; the results consistently showed a direct correlation between US characteristics and tumor angiogenesis associated with malignancy progression [8-12]. In light of these findings, we conducted a prospective study to analyze the relationship between contrast kinetics in the tumorous vessels and histological the type of lesion in an attempt to differentiate between a malignant and benign disease.

METHODS

Patients

One-hundred sixty consecutively examined women with clinically and US-verified adnexal lesions who were referred for surgery were prospectively enrolled in the study. The study was conducted between January 2012 and September 2013. The study was approved by institutional review board and bioethics committee; an informed consent was acquired from all subjects before enrollment. The patients were hospitalized due to diagnosis of unilateral or bilateral adnexal lesions in the form of ovarian tumor, suspected solid-cystic adnexal mass, solid tumor, or similar findings. Following gynecological examination, the patients were referred to the ultrasound examination in order to verify the initial diagnosis. Selected parameters of the tumor were studied, and the degree of vascularization of the pathological lesion was analyzed by means of color Doppler. Patients were eligible for inclusion and imaging with CEUS if during initial ultrasound examination presence of unilateral solid mass or solid-cystic lesion with more than 60% of solid component was declared. The only exclusion criteria were pregnancy and general status which did not enable elective surgery. All women meeting the primary inclusion criteria were referred to surgery and treated by means of laparoscopy or laparotomy depending on age, intraoperative histopathology, clinical advancement of the disease and patients general status at surgeon's discretion. Final histologic diagnoses were obtained for all lesions included in this study and used as reference.

Ultrasound Evaluation and Image Acquisition

Ultrasound examination started with transvaginal and transabdominal real-time grayscale examination of the pelvis, followed by transvaginal color and spectral Doppler US examination of the pelvic mass or masses. The pelvic masses were examined systematically and in a prespecified manner. At two-dimensional real-time US, each mass was classified as follows according to International Ovarian Tumor Analysis (IOTA) Group [13] criteria: 1). a unilocular cyst (a single cyst without septa and without solid parts or papillary excrescences); 2). a multilocular cyst (a cyst with at least one septum but no solid parts or papillary excrescences), 3). a unilocular solid cyst (a single cyst containing solid parts or papillary excrescences but no septa), 4). a multilocular solid cyst (a cyst with at least one septum and solid parts or papillary excrescences), 5). a solid tumor (a tumor with solid components in 60% or more of the tumor). The maximum diameter and volume of the tumor were further measured.

All tumors were examined thoroughly with power Doppler. Each woman contributed only one tumor to the study, thus, if applicable, the tumor with the greatest number of vessels was chosen. A vessel was defined as a separate colored area typical of a blood vessel.

The contrast agent (Levovist Schering AG, Germany) was administered as a bolus 400mg/ml during approximately 10 seconds. All patients were examined at the same B-mode and Color-Doppler settings of ultrasound device (Acuson 128 XP10 device with 7.5 MHz endovaginal probe). The examined area covered the entire adnexal mass or, if the entire lesion was too large, the selected cross-section of its solid part.

In order to standardize the analyzed cross-sections, we visualized the same three morphologically characteristic components of every tumor on grayscale images. Sensitivity was set to the optimal level to visualize small vessels but to avoid noise artifacts.

To assure the reproducibility and to avoid potential discrepancies in the device settings all the examinations and measurements with CEUS were carried out by one physician (MS).

Image Analysis and Endpoints Definitions

Four-minute video clips were recorded and then analyzed offline. Late-phase microvascular imaging projections were reconstructed with Color Quantifier software (CQ, Kinetic Imaging Ltd.) and analyzed to improve lesion detectability. These maximum-intensity projection images depict the overall vascularity of selected regions of interest (ROIs).

The ROI was manually selected to cover the entire mass on the harmonic image. The gray scale intensity of the signals inside the selected ROI were analyzed, and the contrast enhancement time-intensity curves for each tumor were constructed, plotted and analyzed with the CQ Software. The time-intensity curves were normalized by subtracting the mean preinjection (baseline) intensity value from each intensity level (Figure 1).

After that, the following parameters were assessed: 1). The fractional Color Doppler Area (%CDA) was determined for a fixed ROI within each image and defined as the percentage of colored pixels in the given ROI; 2). The time to peak was defined as the time from injection to the peak intensity (T_{MAX}-T_{CON}); 3).

The wash-out time was defined as the time between the peak intensity and the point corresponding to the return to the baseline (T_{END}-T_{MAX}); 4). The Area Under Curve (AUC) was calculated from the arrival of the contrast agent, defined as the point of the increase in image intensity greater than 10% above the baseline to the end of the wash-out period. Additionally, we introduced the S parameter corresponding to the area under the curve and being the definite integral in the following form:

$$S = \int_0^{T^*} F_{\%CDA}(t)dt,$$

where T* is the upper limit of the integration (common to all analyzed plots in some cases). This parameter optimally estimates the results of examination as the value of S is a joint parameter and as such is less susceptible to the fluctuations of particular values of the %CDA function.

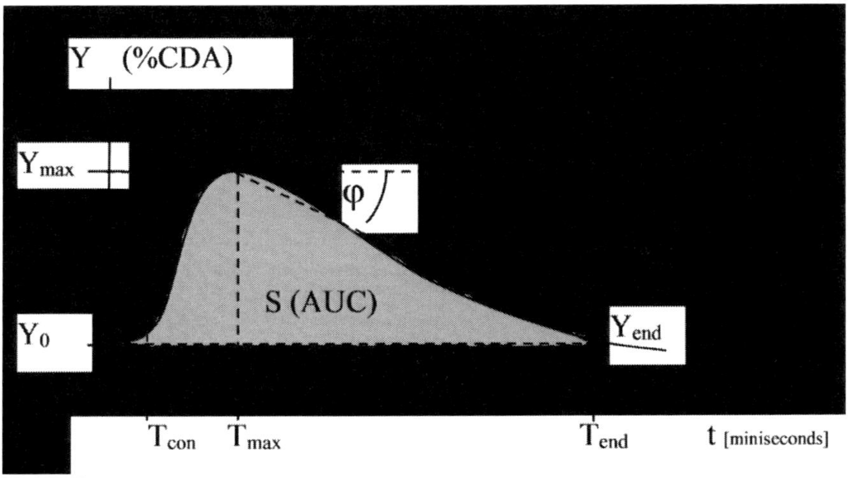

[GRAPH].

%CDA, fractional Color Doppler Area; AUC, Area Under Curve; Tcon, Time point estimate indicating contrast administration.

Figure 1. The time-intensity curve illustrating characteristic sequence of changes taking place during color-enhanced examination.

STATISTICAL ANALYSIS

Mean values along with standard deviations (SD) of selected parameters were calculated. Mann-Whitney U-test was used to compare the variance of acquired contrast kinetics parameters in benign versus malignant lesions analysis. To check if the %CDA maximum values (Y_{max}) were normally distributed Shapiro-Wilk test were employed.

Consequently, the parametric Cochrane-Cox test for unequal variances was used to compare mean values of this variable in studied groups (the hypothesis of variance equality was rejected by the Snedecor F test at $p=0.003$). In the remaining cases the non-parametric Mann-Whitney test was used for intergroup comparisons.

The results were considered significant at two sided p-value <0.05. Statistical analyses were carried out using the statistical package IBM SPSS Statistics 20 (SPSS, Chicago, IL).

RESULTS

Overall, 160 patients, aged between 18 and 90 years, met the enrollment criteria and were qualified to surgery of adnexal lesions. Mean age of the studied group was 56.0±14.5 years. From the initial group, 84 patients were qualified to imaging with CEUS on the basis of strict inclusion criteria. Figure 2. Baseline characteristics of patients and tumors are delineated in Table 1. Serous cystadenocarcinomas (n=73), mucinous cystanedomas (n=22), ovarian metastases (n=18) and benign tumors (n=21) were most commonly occurring tumors and allowed parameters variance testing in the image analyses. Patients with malignant tumors were older (54.5±14.3) than those with benign lesions (45.6±17.2); this difference, however did not reach statistical significance (p=0.06); the remaining characteristics were well balanced between the two groups as confirmed by Mann-Whitney U-test.

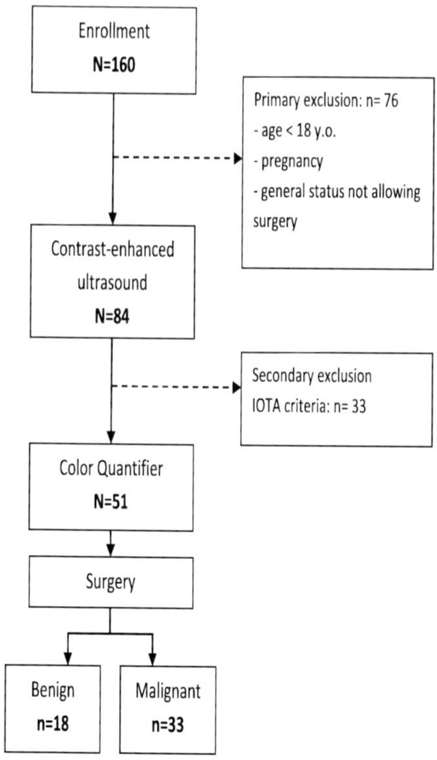

[PTS FLOW].

Figure 2. Study design. IOTA, International Ovarian Tumor Analysis.

Table 1.

Benign lesions (n = 21)	Malignant lesions (n = 139)
	serous cystadenocarcinoma (n = 73)
	mucinous cystadenocarcinoma (n = 22)
	metastatic carcinoma (n = 18)
	germ – cell carcinoma (n = 10)
fibroma (n = 20)	clarocellular ovarian carcinoma (n = 5)
teratoma (n = 1)	small – cell carcinoma (n = 3)
	endometrioid carcinoma (n = 2)
	sarcoma (n = 2)
	squamous carcinoma (n = 2)
	Brenner tumor (n = 1)
	undifferentiated carcinoma (n = 1)

Color Quantifier analysis was performed in 51 pts (33 malignant vs 18 benign) based on secondary inclusion criteria. Figure 2. A diagnostic time-intensity curve with a clearly identifiable start and peak was obtained in all participants (Figure 3). The shape of the obtained curves (Figure 3C and Figure 3D) as well as the selected parameters differed significantly in the benign and malignant tumors evaluation. Mean values and SDs for the indices measured are shown in Table 2.

In the analysis of the time-intensity curves, both the baseline and maximum color Doppler intensities (Figure 3A and Figure 3B), as well as the absolute and relative increases in color Doppler intensity, were significantly higher ($p<0.0001$) in malignant tumors than they were in benign tumors (Table 2). The arrival time of the contrast agent was significantly shorter in malignant tumors than it was in benign tumors ($p<0.0001$). A significant difference in S-parameter, corresponding to the area under curve on the time-intensity chart, between malignant and benign tumor was found as well, with the strongest correlation between S and initial- and peak-intensity %CDA, and was chosen for further analyses (Figure 4A and Figure 4B).

The analysis of empiric distributions of S parameter in the compared groups of tumors (Figure 5) suggests that none of the benign tumors had $S > 90$, which in turn was characteristic for the malignant tumors. Interestingly, malignant tumors fit within $0<S<30$ range markedly less frequently than the benign lesions. The relative prevalence of benign ovarian tumors fitting within this range of S parameter was 11/18 = 0.61, as compared to 6/33 = 0.18 in the case of malignant tumors (Odds Ratio [OR] = 3.36).

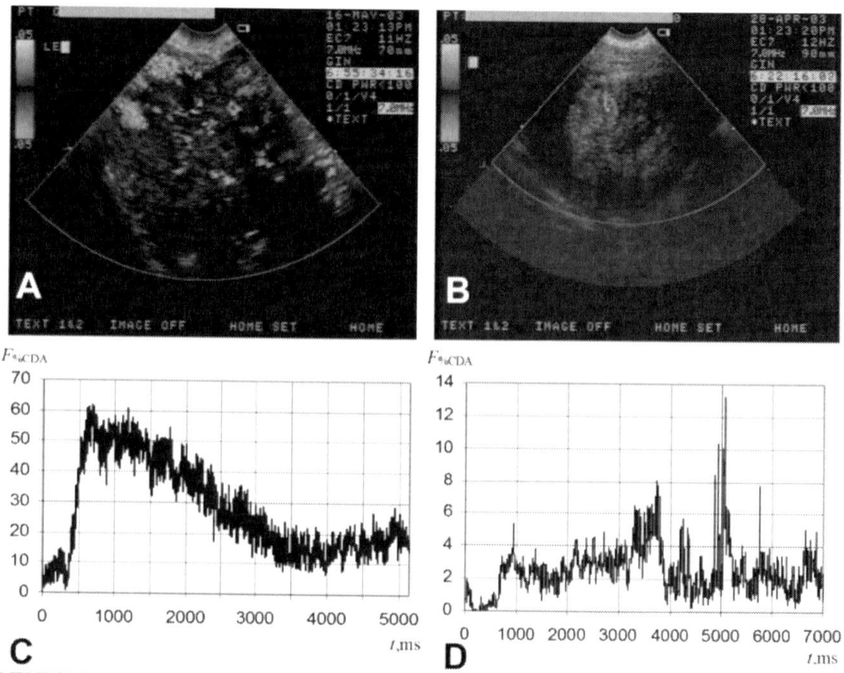

[BENIGN vs MALIGNANT].

Figure 3. Comparison of contrast enhanced ultrasound images in malignant (A) and benign (B) lesions. Contrast kinetics summary in malignant (C) and benign (D) lesions.

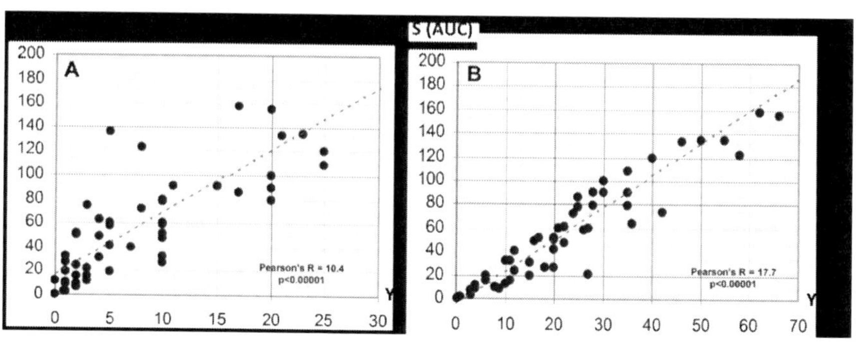

Figure 4. A-linear correlation chart of the S-parameter and Y_0; B-linear correlation chart of the S-parameter and Y_{MAX}; Both charts demonstrate strong statistically significant linear correlation.

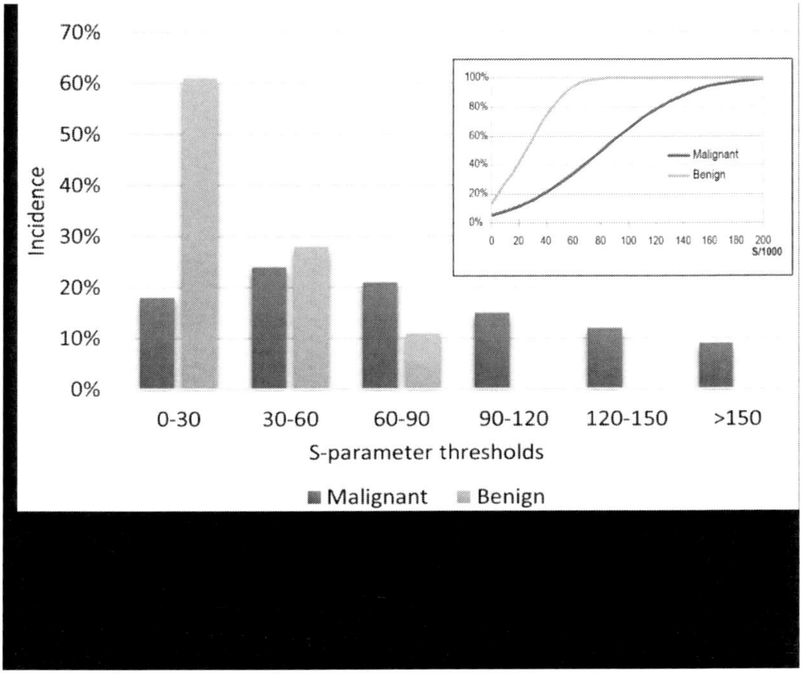

[S-THRESHOLDS AND PROBABILITY].

Figure 5. Distribution of malignant and benign lesions depending on the value of S parameter. Right upper panel shows the probability curves allowing probability inference at given value of the S-parameter to predict the malignant or benign character of the lesion.

Table 2. Comparison of the studied contrast kinetics in benign and malignant subgroups

	Benign lesions (n=18)	Malignant lesions (n=33)
%CDA0	4.27±5.30	10.9±8.4
%CDAMAX	11.3±8.8	31.3±16.9
S (AUC)	25.0±22.7	80.5±50.6

*Cochrane-Cox test. %CDA, fractional Color Doppler Area; AUC, area under curve.

Further analysis revealed that the prevalence of benign tumors within 0<S<30 range is significantly higher than the prevalence of malignant tumors (u=3.12, p<0.002). No significant intergroup differences in prevalence were observed with regards to 30<S<60 and 60<S<90 ranges (p>0.05).

Probability curves at different risk thresholds were further constructed by plotting probability of diagnosis against the value of S-parameter (Figure 5. Right upper panel) Curves indicate that smaller the value of the S-parameter the higher the probability of benign character of the lesion.

DISCUSSION

Final diagnosis of an adnexal mass is based on histopathological examination. However prompt differentiation between benign and malignant character of the lesion before the surgical sampling is of great importance in order to select proper time, place and type of surgery. Intravascular contrast agents increase the intensity of Doppler signals. Thus, they are expected to allow better detection of blood flow in small, deep vessels and this in turn improves the ability to differentiate between areas of normal and abnormal perfusion. Several observational studies have investigated the role of contrast enhanced US (CEUS) in the diagnosis of ovarian tumors with the results consistently showing direct correlation between US characteristics and tumor angiogenesis, in turn associated with malignancy progression [8-12]. It is expected that these differences occur because of the complex and tangled arrangement of the microvascularity and overall increased vascularity within malignant ovarian tumors [14].

The main findings of the present report are that: 1). CEUS is reliable tool, allowing for distinction between malignant and benign pelvic lesions; 2). Neovascularization is a predictor of malignancy; 3). CEUS parameters: shape of the intensity-time curve; %CDA, and AUC (S parameter) correlate linearly with the histological type of the tumor and S-parameter may help in the differentiation between malignant and benign tumors.

International guidelines recommend the use of transvaginal US as the modality of first choice in patients with a suspicious isolated ovarian mass. The extent, however, to which these techniques are reliable and reproducible remains a matter of debate. The accuracies of gray scale sonography and color Doppler imaging for distinguishing malignant from benign tumors range from 80% to 83% and 35% to 88%, respectively [15, 16]. On the other hand, results of a meta-analysis provide scientific evidence that sonographic techniques employed in combination (gray scale morphologic assessment with tumor vascularity imaging) offer significantly better accuracy in ovarian lesion characterization than Doppler arterial resistance measurements, color Doppler flow imaging, or gray scale morphologic information alone [17].

Most physicians are afraid of missing a cancer diagnosis and classify a tumor as malignant at the slightest suspicion of malignancy. Thus, improving specificity without sacrificing sensitivity is one of the main goals of this technology. In this paper one patient was diagnosed false positively based on S-parameter value contributing to the final positive predictive value of 98%.

Use of a contrast agent ascertains more accurate insight of the vascular anatomical relations by enhancement of the signal strength from power Doppler ultrasound, thus enabling dynamic detection of tissue flow of both the macro and microvasculature [18]. This was demonstrated to be particularly valid in solid tumors, in which this enhancement has allowed visualization of higher number of vessels and color pixel densities in malignant than in benign lesions [14, 19-23]. In malignant lesions several specific parameters of neovascularization were universally seen in this study: 1). large diameter with spiral course of the vessel; 2). numerous sharp flexures; 3). irregular ramifications and anastomoses; 3). arteriovenous shunts; 4). lack of gradual narrowing of the vessel; 5) finally, lack of radial penetration of the lesion. Detectable prominent vessels can be seen commonly in benign lesions as well. On the other hand, the morphology and the pattern of vessels distribution and course in benign lesions, including peripheral location within the tumor, straight or slightly spiral course, gradual narrowing, numerous regular ramifications, and eventually higher resistance indices at Color Doppler examination are usually distinguishable from those in malignant tumors. The current report demonstrates at largest possible scale that the evaluation of ovarian tumors based on Color Doppler technique enables determining the qualitative parameters of the dynamic flow in the tumorous vessels. Low values of resistance and pulsatility indices observed within the tumor most commonly reflect the processes of angiogenesis. Therefore, neovascularization may, indeed, be considered a marker of malignancy with the differential diagnosis based on the Doppler assessment of blood perfusion potentially improving the prognostic value of the diagnostic methods employed.

My study with contrast agent also indicate that contrast reaches a peak intensity (%CDA) more rapidly in malignant than in benign tumors and that it persists longer in the malignancies. The former is potentially explained by the rapid flow through arteriovenous shunts and the latter by contrast agent deposition in dilated or blind-ending vessels. Indeed, the brightness of the Power Doppler signal and the volume of recognizable vascular areas increased dramatically in each tumor after contrast agent administration.

In addition, the number of recognizable vessels remained significantly higher in malignant when compared to benign lesions both before and after contrast agent administration. The findings are in line with those obtained by Orden et al. who similarly concluded that each of selected parameters: baseline and maximum power Doppler intensities, duration of the effect and finally the area under the curve significantly correlated with the malignant progression of the disease [8]. The contrast agent uptake time in this study was significantly shorter in malignant than in benign lesions; this could be caused by the high-velocity flow through the arteriovenous shunts that are typically found in malignant neovascularization. The initial arrival of contrast agent results in an excessive widening of color areas, an effect referred to as 'blooming' and is likely to be more pronounced in carcinomas with excessive vasculature [24, 25]. On the other hand, Marret et al. declared that wash-out time of the contrast agent was the parameter that performed the best at predicting malignancy (OR, 1.07; 95% CI, 1.04–1.11; $p < 0.001$), with sensitivity of 96% and specificity of 98% [9]. In this study I used the prespecified parameter S corresponding to intensity-time AUC. It was designed as surrogate measure of both peak enhancement intensity %CDA and wash-out times, and thus, corroborates the estimates from peak intensity %CDA at different time frames of contrast effect. In the same time it does not rely on %CDA fluctuations and different layers of the tumors vasculature alone.

It seems that the most significant clinical application of the data presented would be to develop a high-specificity transvaginal technique for selected difficult to differentiate small solid or cystic-solid tumors with neoangiogenesis and decreased or overexpressed Levovist uptake.

LIMITATIONS

Ovarian angiogenesis and neovascularization may comprise physiologic changes in normal adnexal tissue, especially during premenopausal period. Thus, this physiologic vascular development must be differentiated from pathologic vessels related to malignancy. This study demonstrated high positive predictive value, thus limiting the false positive diagnoses. Accordingly, not the neovascularization itself, but particular vessel's characteristics, which in turn could be obtained by means of CEUS exclusively, have driven those results. Additionally, because the treatment of benign lesions with suspicious morphology consist of surgical resection, these false-positive results would not affect the patients' management protocols. Results of the single-center/single operator study are preliminary and should be interpreted with caution.

The differentiation between malignant and benign character of the lesion is operator dependent, with numerous factors contributing to the final diagnosis. Before definitive conclusions can be drawn, the accuracy and clinical applicability of CEUS large scale comparative studies with diverse diagnostic tools are needed.

Conclusion

The accuracy of the method is higher than that of grey-scale sonography in preoperative differentiation of benign and malignant adnexal tumors. However, further investigation is needed to confirm these findings.

Conflict of interest: I confirm that this paper content has no conflict of interest.

Disclosure: Author do not have any relevant conflict of interest to disclose.

References

[1] American College of Obstetricians and Gynecologists (ACOG). Management of adnexal masses. Washington (DC): American College of Obstetricians and Gynecologists (ACOG); 2007 Jul. 14 p. (*ACOG practice bulletin; no. 83*).

[2] Dodge, J. E., Covens, A. L., Lacchetti, C., Elit, L. M., Le, T., Devries-Aboud, M., Fung-Kee-Fung, M., Gynecology Cancer Disease Site G. Management of a suspicious adnexal mass: a clinical practice guideline. *Curr. Oncol.* 2012;19:e244-257.

[3] D'Arcy, T. J., Jayaram, V., Lynch, M., Soutter, W. P., Cosgrove, D. O., Harvey, C. J., Patel, N. Ovarian cancer detected non-invasively by contrast-enhanced power Doppler ultrasound. *BJOG* 2004;111:619-622.

[4] Cohen, L. S., Escobar, P. F., Scharm, C., Glimco, B., Fishman, D. A. Three-dimensional power Doppler ultrasound improves the diagnostic accuracy for ovarian cancer prediction. *Gynecol. Oncol.* 2001;82:40-48.

[5] Fleischer, A. C., Wojcicki, W. E., Donnelly, E. F., Pickens, D. R., Thirsk, G., Thurman, G. B., Hellerqvist, C. G. Quantified color Doppler

sonography of tumor vascularity in an animal model. *J. Ultrasound Med.* 1999;18:547-551.

[6] Stewart, L., Advanced Ovarian Cancer Trialists G. Chemotherapy for advanced ovarian cancer. Advanced Ovarian Cancer Trialists Group. *Cochrane Database Syst. Rev.* 2000:CD001418.

[7] Engel, J., Eckel, R., Schubert-Fritschle, G., Kerr, J., Kuhn, W., Diebold, J., Kimmig, R., Rehbock, J., Holzel, D. Moderate progress for ovarian cancer in the last 20 years: prolongation of survival, but no improvement in the cure rate. *Eur. J. Cancer* 2002;38:2435-2445.

[8] Orden, M. R., Jurvelin, J. S., Kirkinen, P. P. Kinetics of a US contrast agent in benign and malignant adnexal tumors. *Radiology* 2003;226:405-410.

[9] Marret, H., Sauget, S., Giraudeau, B., Brewer, M., Ranger-Moore, J., Body, G., Tranquart, F. Contrast-enhanced sonography helps in discrimination of benign from malignant adnexal masses. *J. Ultrasound Med.* 2004;23:1629-1639; quiz 1641-1642.

[10] Testa, A. C., Ferrandina, G., Fruscella, E., Van Holsbeke, C., Ferrazzi, E., Leone, F. P., Arduini, D., Exacoustos, C., Bokor, D., Scambia, G., Timmerman, D. The use of contrasted transvaginal sonography in the diagnosis of gynecologic diseases: a preliminary study. *J. Ultrasound Med.* 2005;24:1267-1278.

[11] Fleischer, A. C., Lyshchik, A., Jones, H. W., Jr., Crispens, M., Loveless, M., Andreotti, R. F., Williams, P. K., Fishman, D. A. Contrast-enhanced transvaginal sonography of benign versus malignant ovarian masses: preliminary findings. *J. Ultrasound Med.* 2008;27:1011-1018; quiz 1019-1021.

[12] Enakpene, C. A., Omigbodun, A. O., Goecke, T. W., Odukogbe, A. T., Beckmann, M. W. Preoperative evaluation and triage of women with suspicious adnexal masses using risk of malignancy index. *J. Obstet. Gynaecol. Res.* 2009;35:131-138.

[13] Timmerman, D., Valentin, L., Bourne, T. H., Collins, W. P., Verrelst, H., Vergote, I., International Ovarian Tumor Analysis G. Terms, definitions and measurements to describe the sonographic features of adnexal tumors: a consensus opinion from the International Ovarian Tumor Analysis (IOTA) Group. *Ultrasound Obstet. Gynecol.* 2000;16: 500-505.

[14] Menna, S., Di Virgilio, M. R., Burke, P. [Ultrasonography contrast media Levovist and power Doppler in the study of the breast. Methodology, vascular morphology and automatic enhancement

quantification with wash-in and wash-out curves]. *Radiol. Med.* 1999; 97:472-478.

[15] Buy, J. N., Ghossain, M. A., Sciot, C., Bazot, M., Guinet, C., Prevot, S., Hugol, D., Laromiguiere, M., Truc, J. B., Poitout, P., et al. Epithelial tumors of the ovary: CT findings and correlation with US. *Radiology* 1991;178:811-818.

[16] Reles, A., Wein, U., Lichtenegger, W. Transvaginal color Doppler sonography and conventional sonography in the preoperative assessment of adnexal masses. *J. Clin. Ultrasound* 1997;25:217-225.

[17] Kinkel, K., Hricak, H., Lu, Y., Tsuda, K., Filly, R. A. US characterization of ovarian masses: a meta-analysis. *Radiology* 2000; 217:803-811.

[18] Cosgrove, D. Ultrasound contrast agents: an overview. *Eur. J. Radiol.* 2006;60:324-330.

[19] Kettenbach, J., Helbich, T. H., Huber, S., Zuna, I., Dock, W. Computer-assisted quantitative assessment of power Doppler US: effects of microbubble contrast agent in the differentiation of breast tumors. *Eur. J. Radiol.* 2005;53:238-244.

[20] Huber, S., Helbich, T., Kettenbach, J., Dock, W., Zuna, I., Delorme, S. Effects of a microbubble contrast agent on breast tumors: computer-assisted quantitative assessment with color Doppler US--early experience. *Radiology* 1998;208:485-489.

[21] Fleischer, A. C., Lyshchik, A., Jones, H. W., 3rd, Crispens, M. A., Andreotti, R. F., Williams, P. K., Fishman, D. A. Diagnostic parameters to differentiate benign from malignant ovarian masses with contrast-enhanced transvaginal sonography. *J. Ultrasound Med.* 2009;28:1273-1280.

[22] Fleischer, A. C., Lyshchik, A., Andreotti, R. F., Hwang, M., Jones, H. W., 3rd, Fishman, D. A. Advances in sonographic detection of ovarian cancer: depiction of tumor neovascularity with microbubbles. *AJR Am. J. Roentgenol.* 2010;194:343-348.

[23] Guazzaroni, M., Cossu, E., Danese, V., Montanaro, M., Simonetti, G. [Use of SHU 508 A Levovist contrast media in the characterization of solid lesions of the breast]. *Radiol. Med.* 1998;96:35-41.

[24] Forsberg, F., Liu, J. B., Burns, P. N., Merton, D. A., Goldberg, B. B. Artifacts in ultrasonic contrast agent studies. *J. Ultrasound Med.* 1994; 13:357-365.

[25] Orden, M. R., Gudmundsson, S., Kirkinen, P. Intravascular ultrasound contrast agent: an aid in imaging intervillous blood flow? *Placenta* 1999; 20:235-240.

In: Psychoneurocybernetic Conquest ... ISBN: 978-1-63483-272-4
Editor: Rudolf Klimek

Chapter 5

How Let a Man be Born at His Own Due Time

***Marek Klimek*[1] *and Rudolf Klimek*[2,*]**

[1]Jagiellonian University, Cracow, Poland

[2]Fertility Centre Cracow, Cracow, Poland

Abstract

Both fetus and mother in the last 3-4 days of pregnancy rapidly adapt themselves to delivery and to sudden child's adaptation for postnatal life. Labor which starts one week before its own individual term (preterm) as well as delayed due to disturbance of it's initiation (postponed pregnancy) is possible in the large six-week normal range ($37^{0}/_{7}$ – 43 $^{2}/_{7}$ weeks), which is too big for obstetrical management to estimate the expected date of delivery only by statistical methods. Fetal growth means increase in the size of any of its parts occurring in the process of gestational maturation simultaneously with the mother's adaptation to the labor. New computer-aided ultrasonography method with enzymatic monitoring of advanced pregnancy (≥ 28 weeks) enables to specify the kind of fetal growth rate (fast, regular, slow) and therefore to determine birth-date and newborn's state. The maturity level can be evaluated immediately after labor through obligatory direct assessment of just six of the many possible newborn features: position of the limbs, elbow angle, its mobility, breast nipple, plantar creases and lanugo. The condition of the

* Corresponding author: Prof. Rudolf Klimek, e-mail: mmklimek@cyfronet.pl, phone: +48601547436; fax: +48-12 4225684.

newborn depends mainly on its gestational environment and thus testifies to its mother's health. The progress in neonatology and anesthesiology obscure the iatrogenic labors, which begin at the time improper for individual childbirth, especially due to induction of labor very often instrumental. Reprogramming of ultrasonography biometry and revitalizing of enzymatic monitoring of pregnancies, there is a moral imperative to evaluate fetal maturity of newborn infants immediately after their deliveries. From ethical and medical reasons medicine which is focused only on pathology does not fulfill the requirements of the modern perinatology, which points to the necessity of using the entire human knowledge and does not allow changing physiological events into pathological ones. Both the prophylaxis of premature labors (which belongs to pathology) and non-interference with natural gestational processes (physiology) through unnecessary labor induction or cesarean section at a time improper for individual pregnancy are more important than treatment of premature infants and any prevention of cancers.

Keywords: Biocybernetics, childbirth, fetal maturity, maturity index, oxytocinase, Naegel's rule, newborn maturity, obstetrical carcinogenesis.

ABBREVIATIONS

USG	ultrasonography
EDD	expected date of delivery
F	fast
R	average
S	slow
K	Klimek's maturation index
BPD	Biparietal Diameter
FL	Femur Length

INTRODUCTION

Both fetus and mother in the last 3-4 days of pregnancy undergo rapid pre-labor changes necessary to delivery and sudden child's adaptation to postnatal life [1-10]. Labor which starts one week before its own individual term (preterm) as well as delayed due to disturbance of its initiation (postponed pregnancy) is possible in the large six-week normal range ($37^0/_7$ – $43\ ^2/_7$ weeks). At the beginning of this period the increase in morbidity and mortality is caused not only by labors of multifetal pregnancies, but mainly by lack of help necessary for undiagnosed true preterm births. Reversibly, at the end of the norm (≥ 41st week) premature induction in over ten percent of labors causes' iatrogenic prematurity because of statistical, not individual postdates. Thus obstetricians cannot equally relate the same calendar week of those fetuses, which will indeed be born during this period (e.g., 41st or 43rd), because a preterm birth can occur even at 42nd week just as a post term birth is possible at 38th week owing to failed feto-maternal mechanism of labor initiation.

Unfortunately in contemporary clinical practice even the most sophisticated ultrasonography (USG) imaging equipment fails to provide in advanced pregnancy more accurate information relating to individual birth date than Naegele's Rule (95% confidence interval ± 3 weeks) using only the knowledge of the last menstrual period (LMP) date. In 1985 S. Campbell and co-workers [11] verified Naegele's Rule on 4 000 USG measurements, though their ultrasonography interpretation contained a cardinal error committed, unfortunately, as recently as 1994 [12]. The error lies not in the technologically superior equipment but rather in the application of its programs. Their authors so far have failed to react to critical publications [13-26]. For example, the 40th week on the calendar scale of pregnancy duration may represent for all observed babies only one of three different possibilities: 1) the 40th week for the babies in which delivery is to occur (i.e., birth only for 30% cases), but 2) some babies which had to been delivered e.g., during the 37th week are actually three weeks overdue, while 3) those to be delivered during the 42nd week still have two more weeks prior to birth. Thus pregnancy dating scale which is incorporated in USG programs [27-37] can only provide a statistically probable range of delivery since calendar time is not directly connected to the fetuses' rate of maturity [38-47]. Therefore the object of this paper is to draw also attention to the responsibility of industry for programming their products, if their use could entail medically harmful effects. Instrument, which is advertised as the one that enables to asses fetal age, must not obtain data differing by 1 or 2 weeks in the average values of pregnancy duration, depending on which scale was chosen by the manufacturers. What more a physician who observes closely the development of pregnancy from the last menstrual period will not acquire data for e.g., $42^0/_7$ week, because some calendar scales end at week 40 or 41.

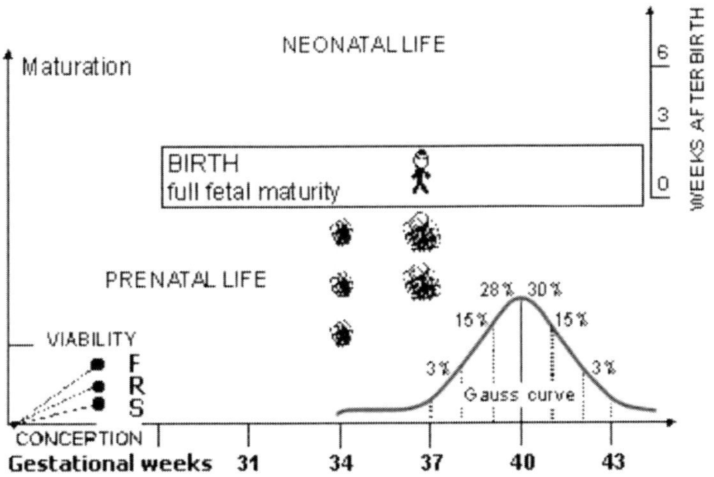

Figure 1. Full fetal maturity among 100 pregnant women at $37^{0/7-6/7}$ gestational week (F - fast, R - average, S - slow).

The six-week period of birth occurrence in a human being is too big for obstetrical management to estimate the expected date of delivery (EDD) only by statistical methods. An increase in instrumental deliveries and lack of progress in lowering the number of premature births associated with increased fetal morbidity and mortality are the consequence of this approach. Fetal growth means increase in the size of any of its parts occurring in the process of gestational maturation simultaneously with the mother's adaptation to the labor. Therefore, new computer-aided ultrasonography method with enzymatic monitoring of advanced pregnancy ($\geq$ 28 weeks) enables to specify the kind of fetal growth rate (fast, regular, slow) and therefore to determine EDD and newborn's state. Enzymatic monitoring of pregnancy is based upon the rule that the constant increase of the oxytocinases level until delivery proves the proper course of pregnancy. In healthy woman the continuous increment of blood oxytocinase level until labor is observed in 81% of cases, slow decreases of levels on several days before labor - in 12%, and it is irregular with variable profile in 7% only [48-51]. As far back as 1930 it has been demonstrated by K. Fekete that the serum of pregnant women was capable of abolishing the uterus-stimulating activity of posterior pituitary extracts. In late forties this feature was linked with enzymes activity called oxytocinase (E. W. Page, K. Semm, E. Werle, G. Effkeman, A. Hevelke, K. Buthmann), but the obtained results have not been adapted in clinical practice. In 1957 H. Tuppy and H. Nesvadba described the principles of chemical assay of the enzyme.

They used as substrate L-cystine-di-ß-naphtylamide indicating erroneously a 1% concentration of solution of sodium nitrate instead of 0,1% what precluded the determination of oxytocinase. In 1961 R. Klimek and M. Pietrzycka revised the methodical error and made the first attempt at establishing an international unit of enzyme activity: μmol/l/min [50]. The following years brought an increasing interest in assessment of aminopeptidase activity in obstetrics (B. Berde, J. Berhard, P. Fylling, G. Graff, T. Hashimoto, H. Kleiner, R. Klimek, S. E. H. Melander. Z. B. Miller, W. Muller-Hartburg, A. P. M. van Oudeusden, A. M. Riad, A.M. Rutenburg, G. Ryden, S. Sakamoto, I. Sjoholm, E.E. Smith, F. Sorm, M. A. Titus, P. Wilken et al.). Unfortunately in 1966 C. Babuna and E. Yenen published a wrong study on the modification of the original chemical assessment of oxytocinase [52-53], which in fact hindered investigations of enzyme monitoring in pregnancy. Three years later R.Klimek delivered a paper in which these laboratory mistakes were corrected [54]. Owing to refusing its publication in Am. J. Obstet. Gynecol. (also this journal published earlier his other clinical studies [51,55,56] it was published in a biochemical journal which was rarely available for the clinicians. Finally, the introduction of new methods of pregnancy monitoring, e. g. human placental lactogen, sonography as well as divergences of opinion on oxytocinase application resulted in groundless neglect of the study on cystine-aminopeptidase activity of pregnant women serum.

Oxytocinase and its isoenzymes reflect the present state of the mother, the child and the placenta – the three being inseparable until the labor components of pregnancy. Maternal blood levels of cystine-aminopeptidases show high correlation with the fetal and placental mass as well as the fetal maturity level. The average values of the enzymes are statistically significantly higher ($p<0.001$) already in the 6th month in the pregnancies which ended in $\geq 39^{th}$ week. Also according to auxological laws 30 days before the labor, fast maturating fetuses have statistically significantly highest enzymatic values, which are the most sensitive indicators of the proper development of fetuses. Enzymes levels and the rate of their increases enable to predict the probable birth term with all the more accuracy, the more similar the subsequent values of the enzymatic determinations. Their low level during pregnancy proves the hypothalamic hypo-function and is a pathognomonic symptom in the habitual abortions caused by such insufficiency. Decrease in levels instead of the normal constant increase precedes by several weeks the intrauterine death of the fetus which reaches 70% when untreated in such neuroendocrine gestoses. The object of this summary is to highlight the importance of enzymatic monitoring which serves as the basis of the biochemical diagnostics in all fields of medicine except for obstetrics. This is particularly odd, as the first enzyme used in medicine was the placenta-produced "defensive pregnancy enzyme" discovered by E. Abderhalden [5-7, 21, 57-60].

COMPUTER-AIDED PROGNOSIS OF CHILDBIRTH

The quantum thermodynamics makes possible prediction of the birth term with the accuracy of ±3-4 days. Owing to this we consider premature each end of pregnancy which has place ≥ 1 week before, and post-term if the labor does not occur ≥ 1 week after the individual term. In each of three components of pregnancy (fetus, mother and placenta with the fetal membranes) several days before the birth term there are clinically noticeable changes which enable verification of the clinical prognoses of birth date and the course of labor done with computer-aided method at ≥28 weeks of gestation. Ultrasonography measurements of selected fetal parameters by means of existing devices are exact and precise; it is only their interpretation that is false. What more, when making physical measurement of one of 100 fetuses in 37th week of pregnancy even by means of the best and unfortunately common percentile scales one cannot conclude if the fetus has to be delivering in days or weeks (Figure 1).

Biometric scales of few fetal parameters used in ultrasound devices are not correlated with one another, therefore the result that assessment of fetal age can differ even in average values by 2 weeks depending on the examined parameter e.g., femur length, head or cranium circumference (Table 1).

Table 1. Average pregnancy age according to the Asian (I, II, III) and European (IV,V,VI) scales of BPD (mm) and FL (mm)

BPD (mm)	Average pregnancy age (weeks + days)					
	I	II	III	IV	V	VI
72	28	29	27+2	27+4	27+1	28+6
92	38	42	37	35+4	35+6	37+3
95	-	-	37	39+6	38+3	38+6
FL (mm)	**I**	**II**	**III**	**IV**	**V**	**VI**
52	29	29	28	27+5	27+3	28+1
55	30+3	30	29+3	29	28+5	29
72	-	40+2	39	36+2	36+5	37

It is caused by the fact that it is not the absolute value of the examined parameters nor the postmenstrual pregnancy duration (calendar time), which determine the birth-date and the condition of the newborns, but the constant growth rate of all spatial fetal parameters (developmental time). Every fetus during the period of maturation (developmental time) must acquire a specific amount of maturity quanta sufficient for self-dependent life, also to eliminate many iatrogenic actions. Adjustment of the existing ultrasound devices to the requirements of the modern medical thermodynamics was patented first in Poland and later in Europe (European Patent No 0557831) which not only proves the originality of the method of ultrasonography fetal biometry and birth prognosis with the accuracy of several days but should primarily force the manufacturers and designers of the faulty scales to change forthwith their way of doing things due to the growing hazard for human health [2-5, 61-63].

Under physiological conditions all tested parameters of individual fetus have the same rate of maturity, but using angular growth rate, computer-aided method gives us clear differentiation between measurements of slow and fast maturing fetuses. The same difference of various sets of ultrasound measurements corresponds to different angles, depending on the elapsed time between consecutive exams. Thus, the same absolute increase of measured ultrasonic parameters between serial measurements at the 1st and 2nd examination do not have a distinctive quality, but decisive is the angle at which growth line will take place over a known period of time.

Physicians' error consist in fact that in spite of the proven simplicity of maturity quantization and its expression in point scale, doctors attempt to measure it on the scale of grams or centimeters or - even worse - of gestational days or weeks. However, it is enough to understand the meaning of the technical quantization which differs from physical one by the fact that scale of examined parameters (quantum) is set on macro level in such a way as to make them multiples of a selected measure. By means of an ultrasonography device we take a measurement of biophysical event such as fetal maturation which is object to be quantized. It suffices to compare a measurement made in 37th or later week to any previous examination $\geq$ 28th week. Then even the same absolute increase in an examined parameter during 2-3 weeks enables to divide fetuses into fast (predicted labor in 37th -38th week), regular (predicted labor in 39th -40th week) and slowly (predicted labor in $\geq$ 41st week) maturating once (Figure 2).

Also in spite of the great technological progress in the production of medical instruments and means of communication, they have not been used to the full in medical procedures. 100 years ago the notion of quantum and later time space were introduced but obstetrician still adhere to out-of-date ideas of absolute time and space. Many of them - even if they know modern definitions of preterm and at term labor – continue to assess fetal maturity according to fetal weight or calendar duration of pregnancy and on that premise they act improperly. Everyone should be aware that on both sides of the mean value of the normal pregnancy duration (281st-283rd days, $40^{1}/_{7}$ - $^{3}/_{7}$ weeks) there are two populations of newborns very much alike in their characteristics. Only 2.5% of these newborns have values of mass, length and maturity higher and lower than the range of the norm of the entire human population. It was proven on hundreds of thousands and even millions of observations of pregnancy duration in the whole world! In the meantime, the scales of modern ultrasonography devices do not cover the whole range of the 95% birth occurrence from $37^{0}/_{7}$ to $43^{2}/_{7}$ weeks after the last menstrual period. To make things worse, as the pregnancy progresses in weeks, the mean values of observed ultrasonography measurements are falsely extrapolated or concealed by providing the wide range of standard duration $\geq$ 3 weeks. These obvious arithmetic errors lead to iatrogenic and mediagenic diseases and social deaths. For example, one of the most frequent causes of instrumental deliveries, as well as the continuing worldwide 7-8% pre-maturity rate, is obstetrician's ignorance of the auxological laws, which are so well known from a next human developmental period i.e., sexual maturation. No one predicts the date of menarche (first menstruation) on the basis of the absolute body mass or height but rather of the rate of their increase. Much better off are pediatricians, who observe auxological standards from the birth of every human being. Every child up until the pubertal spurt generally develops in its own canal (range), whose change must be explained in every case. It is worthy of note that puberty is the next developmental stage following fetal maturation. Children which mature sooner have higher growth parameters than their peers, but the duration of their pubertal spurt is shorter and ultimately they grow to lower height. The same situation occurs during pregnancy before fetus reaches full maturity. The average values which determine weight and length of infants whose maturation is the fastest, i.e., those born in 37th week, are lower than in children born in 38th week, while it is only from 39th week that the characteristics of infants born in the following labor weeks are stabilized. Only newborns in 39th week have the distribution of their features closest to the normal. In fetuses which are born naturally but earlier, the prevailing values are lower than the average, while in the most slowly maturating fetuses the situation is reverse.

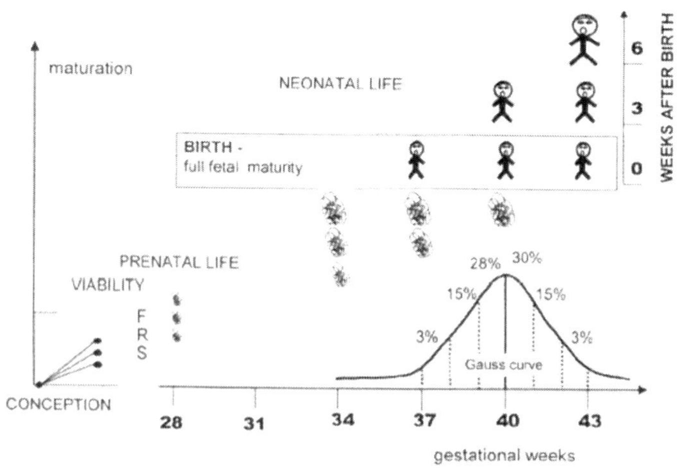

Figure 2. Fetal maturation to the level of viability and self-dependent life.

Thus, the auxological rules must not be disregarded. After all it suffices that in the proper period of pregnancy the obstetrician examines twice the rate of fetal maturation. The data obtained from these examinations allow him to predict the birth-term with the accuracy of several days instead of weeks.

Real and Statistical Birth Term

Everybody knows that he was born on a given one day, while every obstetrician is able to prove that the commencing delivery and its prodromal occur during just two or only three days of profound transformation from pregnancy to labor. Therefore the delivery date has to be estimated with accuracy of ±3 days! Unfortunately, obstetricians single out two days in the calendar pregnancy scale: the 259th day, starting from every fetus is magically considered "mature," and then – somewhat contradictorily – the next day in question is 287th or 294th as the last one to determine maturity. However extensive statistics show that from 287th day of the calendar scale to its 303rd day, there mature over ten percent of slowly developing fetuses. If the physician terminate these pregnancies by inducing labor, in at least several percent of cases he will deliver premature infants. If we consider 100 healthy women (100%) with the same beginning and normal course of pregnancy, 3 of them according to the Gauss curve will deliver in the first and also 3 in the last week of the six-week range of the occurrence of human births within $36^{0}/_{7}$ - $43^{2}/_{7}$ weeks after the last menstrual period, and 30 in each of the middle weeks ($39^{0}/_{7}$ – 40 $^{6}/_{7}$), while only 15 in $38^{0}/_{7}$ – $38^{6}/_{7}$), and in $41^{0}/_{7}$ – $41^{6}/_{7}$ week (see Figure 2).

Table 2. Clinical assessment of Klimek's maturation index in newborn infants

Points	0	1	2
Posture	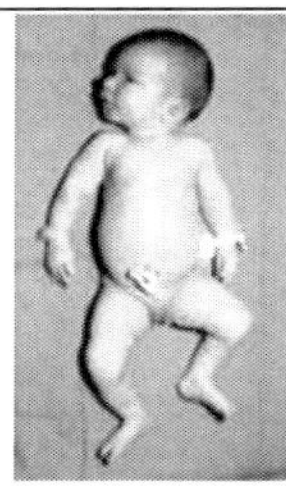	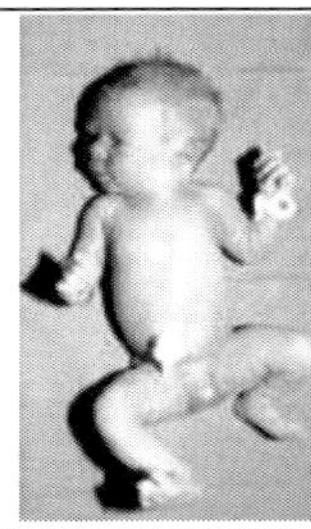	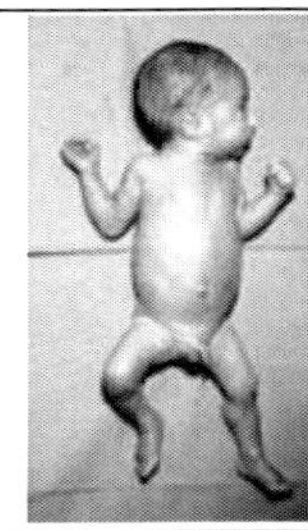
Angle forearm to arm	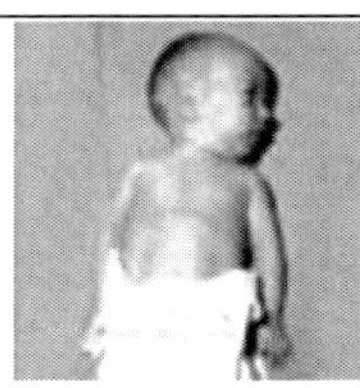 100°-180°	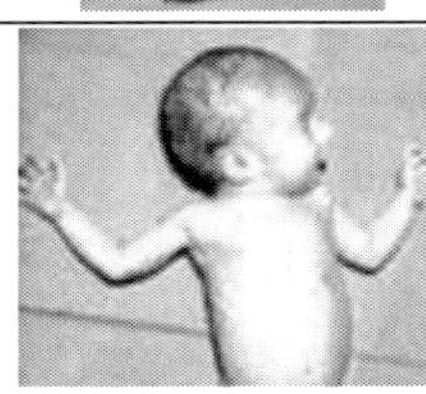 90°-100°	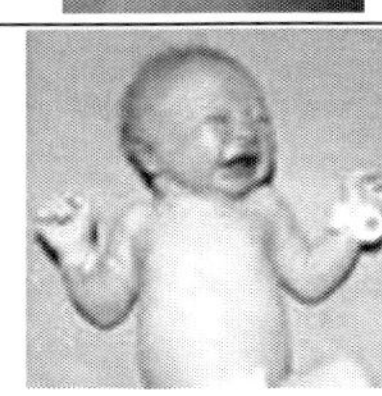 <90°
Pulling an elbow to the body	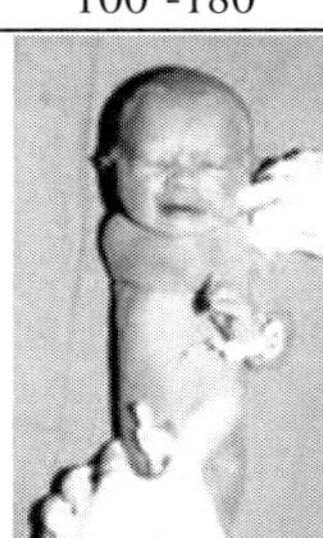	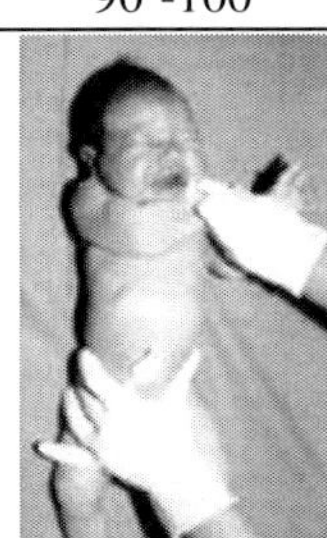	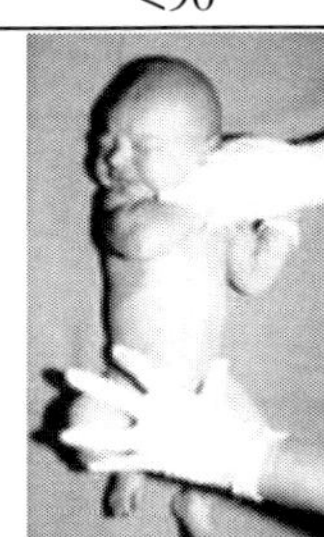
Lanugo	Thinning	single bald areas	mostly bald
Plantar creases	Only on anterior sole	on anterior 2/3 sole	cover entire sole
Breast	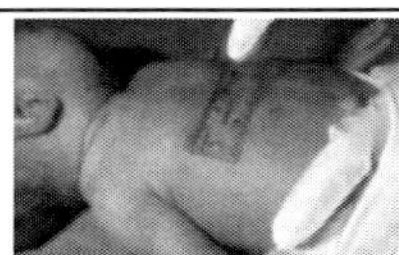 stippled areola bud<3 mm	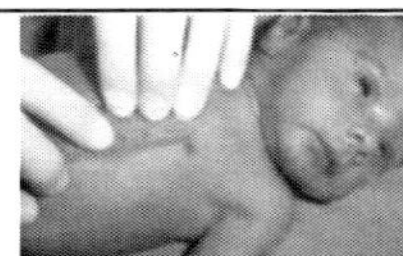 raised areola bud 3-4 mm	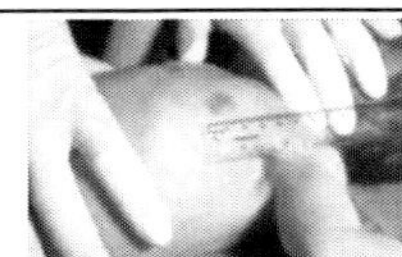 full areola bud > 4mm

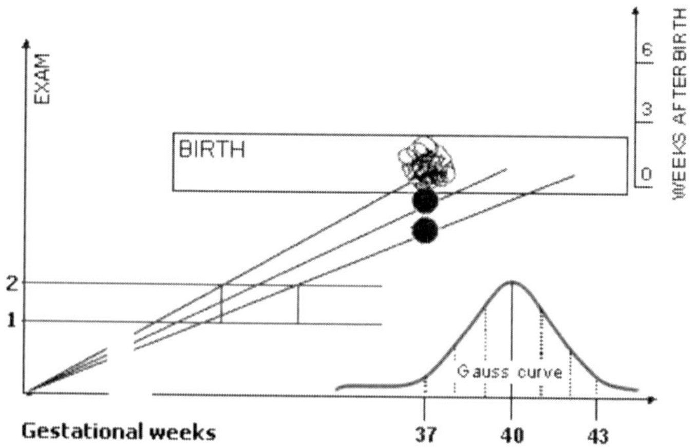

Figure 3. Relative gain of measured parameters (age, mass, size) between I and II exam at different fetal maturation rates (F - fast, A - average, S - slow).

Pregnancy - just as every natural phenomenon (structure or process) - is an individual event whose most important element is fetal maturation of a human being, first to the level of viability, and then to full maturity to self-dependent life. For example, when examine the pregnant women in 40th week, we have to realize that only approximately 30 out of their fetuses are mature for labor and other ones will deliver - unless pregnancy is iatrogenically terminated - after 287th day of physiologic pregnancy $\geq 41^{0}/_{7}$ week. After the 42nd week still 3% of children can be physiologically delivered.

How can one predict in the observed individual pregnant women, in which of the 6 weeks, than labor has to occur?

First of all, it needs to be stressed that ultrasonography measurements of selected fetal parameters by means of existing devices are exact and precise; it is only their interpretation that is false. When making physical measurement of individual fetus only once in advanced weeks of pregnancy one cannot conclude if the fetus has to be delivering in days or weeks (see Figure1).

Fetal maturity is a feature like other measurable fetal material-energetic ones, but also it is information related to distribution and state of mass and energy in developing fetus. At the atomic level each subsequent new indivisible unit (quantum) of fetal maturity appears at a particular time which is inseparable from maturing fetal body. Delivery occurs when a full quanta of fetal maturity has been completed. Thus, accordingly to the quickness of appearance of the consecutive quanta some fetuses are already mature at $37^{0}/_{7}$

postmenstrual week of gestation while the other ones have to mature until $43^2/_7$ (95% of confidence limits).

The maturity level can be evaluated immediately after labor through direct assessment of just six of the many possible newborn features: position of the limbs, elbow angle forearm (100-180°, 90° -100°, <90°); its mobility by pulling an elbow to the middle line of the body; breast nipple development (areola appearance and bud size less than 3-4 mm or more than 4 mm), appearances of plantar creases and lanugo (Table 2).

For each of those features one can allocate from 0 to 2 points, which maximally gives 12 technical quantum points of Klimek's maturation index (K) in newborn infants for the full fetal maturity: 9±1.5 points in the range from 6 to 12 points, while immature newborns have less than 6 points [62-65]. The new method differs from generally known Amiel-Tison's, Dubowitz and Ballard methods in the smaller range of allocated points, and what is more important- the possibility of making the assessment during routine examination of newborn baby immediately after its birth. New index does not take into account weight and fetal age. The obtained values of maturity index K indicate a high statistical correlation with the results of both computer-aided method of advanced pregnancy prediction of full fetal maturity and the actual postnatal method of maturity assessment developed by Ballard [64]. The distribution of the mature newborn according to their K index values was found equal to the statistical and auxological conditioned human birth occurrence [63, 66-69].

CONCLUSION

Modern medical means as ultrasonography devices, cardiotocographs or neonatological incubators from the technical point of view stems from the greatest advances of quantum mechanics, theory of relativity and biocybernetics. Unfortunately, their use in obstetrics sometimes paradoxically leads to iatrogenic morbidity and mortality due to lack of understanding of fetal maturation and relativity of calendar pregnancy duration [70-75]. The condition of the newborn depends mainly on its gestational environment and thus testifies to its mother's health. This is what differentiates modern medical thermodynamics from the labor mechanics of the bygone era of the absolute time and space. Medicine which is focused only on pathology does not fulfill the requirements of the modern perinatology, which points to the necessity of using the entire human knowledge and does not allow to change physiological events into pathological ones. Both the prophylaxis of premature labors (which belongs to pathology) and non-interference with natural gestational processes (physiology) through unnecessary labor induction or cesarean section at a time improper for individual pregnancy are more important than treatment of premature infants [76-84]. From ethical and medical reasons the progress in neonatology and anesthesiology obscure the iatrogenic labors for individual childbirth, especially due to induction of labor very often instrumental. Labor at an improper time is a common obstetrical error, which finds confirmation among others in higher perinatal mortality indexes at preterm labors one week before true individual term, by being consequence of iatrogenic induction of the labor. By means of the existent ultrasonography devices, but taking into account biocybernetics one can made - on the basis of two measurements within ≥2 weeks - not only assess the current maturity, mass, length and gestational age of the child, but also predict those values in the perinatal period. It brings measurable medical, social and financial profits and - most importantly – discards the ethics of reticence on the dangerous dominance of technology over general knowledge. It also reminds the doctors that their first obligation remains the tenet "primum non nocere" [85-90].

There was a time when improper use of cardiotocographs resulted in too much irreversible medical and social damage. The time has come to point one's finger at manufacturers and users who bear the responsibility for similar effects in obstetrical ultrasonography. This is the best way to bring the percentage of prematurity down to the natural limit of 2.5% of all deliveries. Currently, 10-18% of labors are induced prematurely only because the calendar time of pregnancy duration has exceeded 287 or 294 days from the date of the last menstrual period, which additionally is given by the mothers accurate to several days, anyway. The reduction of perinatal mortality – sometimes wrongly ascribed mainly to obstetricians – is primarily an effect of the amazing progress in neonatology. Low birth weight, perinatal mortality and prematurity rate have been even adopted as general social and economic indices of development of entire countries or at least selected territories. Therefore, to bring out the role of obstetricians there in, one should permanently introduce two other clinical criteria: distribution of birth in the range of six-week norm of occurrence in humans and ratio of premature infants to the mature ones at the gestational age [91-95].

After reprogramming of ultrasonography biometry as well as revitalizing of enzymatic monitoring of pregnancies, there is a moral imperative to evaluate fetal maturity of newborn infants immediately after their deliveries. Such individual evaluation of each delivery ought to be performed directly in obstetrical ward not only by routine assessment of the adaptation of the newborn in Apgar scale but also of its fetal maturity according to new index K of fetal maturity, what is particularly important in the case of instrumental deliveries.

REFERENCES

[1] Klimek, M. Psychological aspects of determining the expected date of delivery. *Int. J. Prenat. Perinat. Psychology Medicine*, 1993, 5, 150–155.

[2] Klimek, M. Computer-aided imaging in advanced pregnancy. In: Popkin, D. R. and Peddle L.J. (Eds): Women's Health Today. The Proceedings of the XIV FIGO World Congress, *Montreal Parthenon*, New York-London, 1994, 245-250.

[3] Klimek, M. A Critical Evaluation of Fetal Weight Assessment in Late Pregnancy *Int .J Prenatal and Perinatal Psychology and Medicine*, 1995, 7(1), 17-22.

[4] Klimek, M. Computer-Aided Ultrasonic Fetometry in Advanced Pregnancy *Int.J. Prenatal and Perinatal Psychology and Medicine*, 1995, 7(1), 7-16.

[5] Klimek, M. Medical prognosis versus statistical prediction of birth term In: Klimek, R., Fedor-Freybergh, P., Janus, L., Walas-Skolicka, E. (Eds) A Time to Be Born DREAM Publishing Company 1996, Cracow 9-33.

[6] Klimek, R. Relative duration of human pregnancy and oxytocin therapy. Part I. *Gynecologia*, 1967, 163, 48-53.

[7] Klimek, R. Relative duration of human pregnancy and oxytocin therapy. Part II. Enzymic block. *Gynecologia*, 1967, 167, 54-64.

[8] Klimek, R. Ultrasonography in terms of biological and calendar gestational age. Report F.I.G.O - Study Group on "Assessment of New Technology" DWN DReAM, 1991, Cracow.

[9] Klimek, R. Computerized prediction of fetal birth-weight and birth-date using ultrasound measurements in advanced pregnancy 2nd World Congress of Ultrasound in Ob/Gyn, *Bonn Book of abstracts*, 1992, 119.

[10] Skręt-Magiełło, J; Wicherek, L; Basta, P; et al. RCAS1 decidual immunoreactivity during the cesarean section scar. Deciduosis immune cell presence and activity. *Gin. Obst. Invest.*, 2008, 65, 187-194.

[11] Campbell, S; Warsof, SL; Little, D; Cooper, DJ. Rutine Ultrasound Screening for the Prediction of Gestational Age Obstet. *Gynaecol*, 1995, 65, 613.

[12] Chitty, L.S, Altman, DG; Henderson, A; Campbell, S. Charts of fetal size: 4. *Femur length Brit J Gynecol Obstet*, 1994, 101, 132-5.

[13] Cosmi, EV; Klimek, R; et al. (FIGO Study Group Members) Reccomendations on the use of ultrasound and Doppler technology in clinical obstetrics and gynecology. Int. J. Gynecol. Obstet, 1992, 37, 221-228.

[14] Cosmi, EV; Klimek, R. Philosophy of birth: Natural process or artificial obstetrical procedure? *Int. J. Gynecol. Obstet.*, 1993, 41, 231-232.

[15] Cosmi, EV; Klimek, R; Di Renzo, GC; Kulakov, V; Kurjak, A; Maeda, K; Mandruzzato, GP; Van Gelin, HP; Wladimiroff, J. Prognosis of birth term: recommendations on current practice and overview of new developments *Archiv. Perinat. Med.*, 1997, 3(2), 31-50.

[16] Rzepecka-Węglarz B; Klimek M; Frączek A; Lauterbach R. (2000) Kliniczny sposób oceny dojrzałości noworodka według wskaźnika R.Klimka. (Clinical method of newborn's maturity evaluation according to R.Klimek's index), *Gin. Pol*, 71, 1, 1-7.

[17] Klimek, M; Frączek, A; Klimek, R; Michalski, A. Procedural errors of ultrasound dating of pregnancy using fetal dimensions *Archivo Ostetrica e Ginecologia*, 1993, 2, 1–4.

[18] Klimek, M; Klimek, R; Mazanek-Mościcka, M. Biological diagnosis and prognosis in practical obstetrics Polish J.Gynaec.Invest. 1999, 2, 57-66

[19] Klimek, R. Ultrasonographers contra Leonardo da Vinci. Quo vadis obstetric sonography? *Int. J. Gynecol. Obstet*, 1993, 3, 114-117.

[20] Klimek, R. Birth-term: one day or five weeks. The Proceedings of 2nd World Congress on Labor and Delivery. *The Parthenon Publishing Group*, 1997, 45-49

[21] Klimek, R. (ed.), G.H.Bręborowicz, B. Chazan, K. Czajkowski, R.Dębski, J.Dubčák, P. Fedor-Freybergh, Z.Hájek, K.Kamiński, M.Klimek, J. Krzysiek, R.Lauterbach, S.Lukačín, A. Malarewicz, Z.Maly, L.Marianowski, J.Oleszczuk, T.Pisarski, A. Roztočil, S.Sajdak, A.Skręt, J. Štencl, W. Szymański, J. Wilczyński, V.Unzeitig, Z.Zdebski. Declaration of the Chilbirth in XXI Century, *Cracow. Arch. Perinat. Med.*, 2001, 7(3), 8-14

[22] Mazanek-Mościcka, M; Pabian, W. The Cracow Obstetrical School – main achivements. *Arch. Perinat.* Med. 2001, 7(3), 37-41.

[23] Štembera, Z. Development of the frequency of obstetric operations and perinatal mortality in the Czech Republic, as compared with other countries *Ces. Gynek.*, 1995, 60, 131-138.

[24] Štembera, Z; Holub, J. Hospitalisation during pregnancy-Professional vs. economic aspects *Ces.Gynek.*, 1996, 1, 332-337.

[25] Callen, PW. Ultrasonography in Obstetrics and Gynecology 3rd ed *W. B. Saunders Company*, 1994, Philadelphia.

[26] Klimek, R. Profilaktyczno-terapeutyczne szczepienie przeciwko stanom przedrakowym szyjki macicy. [Prophylactic and therapeutic vaccination against precancerous states of uterine cervix]. *Gin. Prakt.* 2007, 15(2), 36-40.

[27] Hadlock, FP, Deter, Ludwig R. et al. Estimating fetal age *Am. J Obstet. Gyn.*, 1981, 141, 759.

[28] Klimek, R. (ed). Pre–Peri Natal Psycho–Medicine DWN DreAM 1992, Cracow.

[29] Klimek, R. Ultrasound assessment of fetal growth and prediction of birth-date in late pregnancy *Int. J. Prenatal Perinatal Psychology Medicine*, 1973, 5, 1, 1-13.

[30] Klimek, R. Obstetrical interpretation of individual birth at term J.Perinat.Med., *WAPM-Newssletter*, 1998, 26, 69-72.

[31] Merz, A. Ultrasound in Gynecology and Obstetrics: *Text and Atlas G. Thieme*, 1991, New York.

[32] Rossavik, JK. Practical Obstetrical Ultrasound. Stillwater 1st World Publishing Company 1991.

[33] Sabbagha, RE. Diagnostic Ultrasound applied to Obstetrics and Gynecology. 3rd ed. *J. B. Lippincott Company*, 1994, Philadelphia.

[34] Klimek, R. Nuclear magnetic resonance in obstetrics and gynecology. Int. J. Gynecol. Obstet. 1990, 32, 199-205.

[35] Klimek, R. Statistically orientated ultrasound prediction of birth terms as possible iatrogenic event. 8th *Congress of European Association of Gynecologists and Obstetricians*, 1993, Ljubljana, Slovenia: FC 42.

[36] Alexander, GR; Himes, JH; Kaufman, RB; Mor, J; Kogan, M. A United States national reference for fetal growth *Obstet Gynecol.*, 1996, 87(2), 163-8.

[37] Czajkowski, K; Szymański, Eds. Rudolfa Klimka Położnictwo. [R. Klimek's Obstetrics]. RK 2006, Kraków.

[38] Frączek, A; Klimek, M; Klimek, R; Pabian, W. New ultrasound assessment of the fetal weight in advanced pregnancy Pre-Neonatal Medicine, 1998, 3, supll. 161.

[39] Hoseman, H. Normale und abnormale Schwangerschaftsdauer In: Biologie und Pathologie des Weibes. Verlag Urban Schwarzeberg 1952, *Berlin*, 828.

[40] Klimek, M; Frączek, A; Hann, R; Hassan, H; Grzegorek, K. Prospective clinical evaluation of fetal weight gain in late pregnancy by means of computer aided fetometry. *Archivio di Ostetricia e Ginecologia*, 1994, 2, 53-56.

[41] Klimek, M; Frączek, A; Hassan, H; Klimek, R. Computer-aided ultrasound monitoring of fetal therapy with ACTH-depot The Fourth World Congress on Ultrasound in Obst. and Gyn. 1994, *Budapest*, 146.

[42] Klimek, M; Klimek, R; Skotniczny, K; et al. Auxiological relations between prenatal ultrasound and oxytocinase measurements high-risk pregnancies. *J. Prenat. Neonat. Med.*, 2001, 6, 350-55.

[43] Klimek, R. Biological gestational age and its calendar assessment with ultrasound. Part 1, *Physiological Considerations Gynekol. Geburtsh. Rundsch.*, 1992, 32, 95-99.

[44] Klimek, R; Jasiczek, D; Gralek, P; Fedor-Freybergh, P. Cancer – final cellular form of life. *Int. J. Prenat. Perinat. Psychol. Medicine*, 2011, 23, 7-17.

[45] Klimek, R; Klimek, M. Biological gestational age and its calendar assessment with ultrasound. Part 2. Biological–Calendar Scales for Prediction of Birth–date Gynaecol. *Geburst. Rundsch.*, 1992, 32, 159–63.

[46] Klimek, R. Enzymes: The Most Important Markers Of Pregnancy Development J.Early Pregnancy: *Biology and Medicine*, 2000, 4, 219-229.

[47] Klimek, R; Fedor-Freybergh, P; Janus, L; Walas-Skolicka, E. A Time to Be Born. *DREAM Publishing Company, Inc.*, 1996, Cracow.

[48] Klimek, R; Rzepecka, A; Klimekm M; Michalski, A. Enzymatic and ultrasonographic monitoring of pregnancy and prediction of birth-date EAGO-Polish Branch-ISPPM, 1992, Cracow.

[49] Klimek, R; Stanek, J. Comparative prognostic value of serum placental and tissue oxytocinase, alcaline phosphatase and its heat-stable fraction in pregnancy at neuroendocrinological risk *J. Perinat. Med.*, 1976, 4, 234.

[50] Klimek, R; Pietrzycka, M. Biochemische Methode zur Bestimmung der Oxytocinase und Klinische Bewertung. [Biochemical method for the determination of oxytocinase and its clinical value]. *Clin. Chim. Acta*, 1961, 6, 326.

[51] Klimek, R; Drewniak, K; Bieniasz, A. Further studies on the oxytocin-oxytocinase system *Am. J. Obstet. Gynec.*, 1969, 105, 427-32
[52] Babuna, C; Yenen, E. Further studies on serum oxytocinase in pathologic pregnancy *Am. J. Obstet. Gynecol*, 1966, 94(6), 868-75.
[53] Babuna, C; Yenen, E. (1966) Enzymatic determination of placental function. A rapid method *Am J Obstet Gynecol*, 1966, 95(7), 925-34.
[54] Klimek, R. Clinical studies on the balance beetwen isooxytocinases in the blood of pregnant women. *Clin Chim Acta*, 1968, 20, 233-238.
[55] Klimek, R; Bieniasz, A. Studies on the relation between serum oxytocinase and labor *Am. J. Obst. Gynec.*, 1969, 104, 959-963.
[56] Bieniasz, A; Drewniak, K; Klimek, R. Clinical studies on desaminooxytocin *Am J Obstet Gynecol.*, 1967, 98, 535-539.
[57] Klimek, R. Monitoring of Pregnancy and Prediction of Birth–date The Parthenon Publishing Group 1994, London – New York.
[58] Klimek, R; Małolepszy, E. Evaluation of a rapid enzymatic method for determining placental function *Clin. Chim. Acta*, 1969, 24, 349-352
[59] Klimek, R. Computer aided ultrasound monitoring of twin pregnancy 2nd Int.Congress on New Technologies in Reproductive Medicine, Neonatology and Gynecology, Sardynia, book; In: Cosmi E.V. (ed), *Monduzzi Editore Int.Proceedings Div.*, 1999, 97-102.
[60] Klimek, R. The use in obstetrics of quantum theory as well as modern technology to decrease the morbidity and mortality of newborns and mothers during iatrogenic induced delivery *Neuroendocrinology Letters*, 2001, 22, 5-8.
[61] Klimek, R; Frączek, A; Klimek, M. Prognosis of birth term: new developments 1 Inter. Symp. “New Technologies in Reproductive Medicine, Neonatology and Gynecology,” Folgaria 1998, Abstr. R55, *The Parthenon Publ.Group*, 1999, 107-110, New York-London.
[62] Klimek, R. New obstetrical index of newborn maturity.Prenatal and Neonatal Medicine, XVI Inter. Congress The Fetus as a Patient, Fiuggi, Italy In: E.V.Cosmi (ed) The Fetus As A Patient, *Monduzzi Editore S.p. A*, 2000, 61-65.
[63] Klimek, R. Estimation of biological gestational age by corrected Ballard "Maturation rating" World Congress of Perinatal Psychology and Medicine, Cracow; Archivo di Obstetricia e Gynecologia, 1, 25-28, *Int. J. Prenatal Perinatal Studies*, 1992, 4, Suppl.1, 101-110
[64] Ballard, JL; Novak, KK; Weding, K; at al. New Ballard score expanded to include extremely premature infanrts. *J Pediatr*, 1991, 119, 417-23.

[65] Klimek, R; Klimek, M; Rzepecka-Węglarz, B. A new score for postnatal clinical assessment of fetal maturity in newborn infants *Int J. Obst. Gyn.*, 2000, 71, 101-105.

[66] Klimek, R; Lauterbach, R. Posnatal clinical assessment of fetal maturity in new born infants. *Arch. Perinat. Med.*, 2001, 7(3), 19-23.

[67] Klimek, R; Klimek, M; Gralek, P; Jasiczek, D. Causal ACTH-depot therapy during pregnancies following infertility treatment. *Obstetrics Gynecology International*, 2012, Volume 2012, article ID 248926, 7 p.

[68] Klimek, R. Conquering cancer ourselves. New trends in gynecology and obstetrics. *J. Libbey CIC s.r.l; Roma*, 1990, 6 (2), 53-117.

[69] Rzepecka-Węglarz, B. Neonatologic assessment of ultrasonographic and enzymatic estimators of fetal maturity. Doctor's thesis (Polish), Cracow, *Jagiellonian University*, 1999.

[70] Tadeusiewicz, R. Place and Role of Intelligent Systems in Computer Science. *Computer Methods in Materials Science*, 2010, 10 (4), 193-206.

[71] Fedor-Freybergh, PG; Maas, L. Continuity and indivisibility of integrated psychological, spiritual and somatic life processes. *Int. J. Prenat. Perinat. Psychol. Medicine*, 2011, 23, suppl. 1, 135-42.

[72] Hodorowicz, S; Jasiczek, D; Klimek, R; Tadeusiewicz, R; Eds. Rak i niepłodność. Prawda i mity medycyny. [Cancer and infertility. Truth and myth of medicine]. Kraków-Warszawa: Trio 2011.

[73] Jasiczek, D; Kaim, I; Czajkowski, K. Historic discovery of natural thermodynamic cause of cancer. *Neurocrinol. Letters*, 2012, 33(4), 101-11.

[74] Jasiczek, D; Klimek, R; Štencl, J; Tadeusiewicz, R; Tholt, M. Obstetrical prevention of human cancers. *Neuroencrinology Letters*, 2012, 33(2), 118-23.

[75] Hajek, Z; Haakova, L; Kolarik, D; et al. Operative deliveries, professional and economic aspects. *Arch. Perinat. Med.*, 2001, 7(3), 30-32.

[76] Joffe, M; Chapple, J; Paterson, C; et al. What is the optimal caesarean section rate? An outcome based study of existing variation J. *Epid.Comm.Health*, 1994, 48, 406-411.

[77] Klimek, M; Klimek, R; Mazanek-Mościcka M. Preterm birth as an indicator of cancer risk for the mother. *It. J. Gynacol. Obstet.*, 2002, 3, 73-77.

[78] Nielson, TF; Hokegard, KH. Caesarean section and intraoperative surgical complications. *Acta Obstet.Gynec.Scand.*, 1984, 63, 103-108.

[79] Notzon, FC. International differencies on the use of obstetrical interventionas. *J. Amer. Med. Ass.*, 1990, 263, 3286-3291.

[80] Pettiti, DB. Maternal mortality and morbidity in caesarean section *Clin.Obstet.Gynec*. 1985, 28, 763-768.

[81] Srp, B; Velebil, P. Proportion of caesarean section and main causes of maternal mortality during 1978-1997 in the Czech Republic Ces. Gynek., 1999, 64, 219-223

[82] Sachs, BP; Yeh, J; Archers, D; et al. Caesarean section related maternal mortality in Massachusetts 1954-1985, *Obstet. Gynec.*, 1987, 69, 696-700.

[83] Klimek, R; Klimek, M; Jasiczek, D. Immunotherapy of cervical cancer as a biological dissipative structure. *Neuroendocrinology Letters*, 2011, 32(4), 380-88.

[84] Schenker, JG. Ethical dileman in perinatal medicine. Jaypee Brothers Medical Pub. New Delhi 2010.

[85] Schenker, JG. Stress and human reproduction. In: Klimek, R, Ed. *Pre-Peri-Natal Psycho-Medicine*, 1992, DreAM Cracow, p. 77-82.

[86] Klimek, R; Czajkowski, K; Kojs, Z; Szymański, W; Śpiewankiewicz, B. Psychoneurocybernetyczna etiopatogeneza raków. Psychoneurocybernetic etiopathogenesis of cancers. *Curr. Gynecol. Oncol.*, 2013, 11(3), 202-09.

[87] Klimek, R; Kolenda, Z. Carcinogenic entropy. *Curr. Gynecol. Oncol.*, 2013, 11(1), 10-20.

[88] Kurjak, A; Chervenak, FA; Eds. Controversies on the beginning of human life. New Delhi: Jitendar 2008.

[89] Tadeusiewicz, R. New Trends in Neurocybernetics. *Computer Methods in Materials Science.*, 2010, 10(1), 1-7.

[90] Klimek, R. Clinical psychology in terms of ecumenical medicine. *Pre– and Perinatal Psychology Journal*, 1993, 8(2), 119-128.

[91] Yerushalmy, J. Relation of birth weight, gestational age, and the rate of intrauterine growth to perinatal mortality. *Clin Obstet Gynecol.*, 1970, 13(1), 107-29.

[92] Kirkinen, P. Multiple caesarean sections: outcome and complications Brit. *J.Obstet.Gynaec.*, 1988, 95, 778-782.

[93] Klimek, R. Cervical cancer as a natural phenomenon. *Eur. J. Obstet. Gynecol. Reprod. Biol.*, 1990, 36, 221-238.

[94] Khroutski, KS. Forming an evolutionary vector to the Aristotelian Pole of scientific Organicism. Biocosmology-neoAristotelism 2013, Vol. 3(1)

28-52. URL://en.biocosmology.ru/electronic-journal-biocosmology---neo-aristotelism.

[95] Minakami, H; Sato, I. Reestimating date of delivery in multifetal pregnancies. *JAMA*, 1996, 275(18), 1432-4.

In: Psychoneurocybernetic Conquest … ISBN: 978-1-63483-272-4
Editor: Rudolf Klimek

Chapter 6

BIOCYBERNETICS LINKS MEDICINE AND TECHNOLOGY

Ryszard Tadeusiewicz*
Head of Automatic Control and Biomedical Engineering Chair and Director of Biocybernetics Laboratory in AGH University of Science and Technology, Cracow, Poland

ABSTRACT

Development of biological science, including medicine, is really imposing at the beginning of the 21st century, e.g., a prolonging life expectancy of people born in subsequent years. The progress of technology is also extremely fast, performing things which seemed absolutely unachievable a few years ago. However, in reality a peculiar mental "wall" has grown between the two fields of different methodology and different developmental traditions as well as a hermetic, different terminology. Therefore the new branch of science, which is biocybernetics, may help medical doctors and technicians to communicate "discounting the differences," despite that "wall." It is not possible for engineers to learn physiology or for doctors to learn the secrets of mechanics. Nevertheless it is possible to suggest such a description of the considered systems and processes, which will match both biological phenomena and technical devices. The methods of using that description will be equally easy for doctors as for engineers.

* Corresponding author: Prof. Ryszard Tadeusiewicz, Al.Mickiewicza 30, 30-059 Cracow, Poland, e-mail: rtad@agh.edu.pl.

Biocybernetics offers such ways and that is why it can be used as a peculiar "bridge" allowing for overcoming the differences dividing technology from biology and medicine. Due to that it is possible to cross the "wall" dividing the mentioned fields. The key to success is abstraction as an informational method. Thanks to its high level the description created on the basis of biocybernetics can fit both to biology, as well as technology. Such a way of biocybernetic attainment of new knowledge on objects and biological processes has already gained big respect among researchers and is sometimes called an "*experiment in compute*" to resemble traditionally held biological experiments on tissues separated from organisms, called an "*experiment in vitro*" or "*experiment in vivo*." One must claim that biocybernetics is still not a commonly used method supplementing traditional research methods in biology and medicine but it has a chance to become a commonly used procedure.

Keywords: Biocybernetics, biocybernetic model, experimental biology, medicine, abstraction

INTRODUCTION

Development of biological science, including medicine, is really imposing at the beginning of the 21st century. This can be observed in, among other, both a prolonging life expectancy of people born in subsequent years and a diminishing number of deaths for 100,000 people. This statistical data is commonly known and generates great respect. Development and progress of technology is also extremely fast. We send people into space, search the bottom of oceans (Figure 1) and perform things which seemed absolutely unachievable a few years ago.

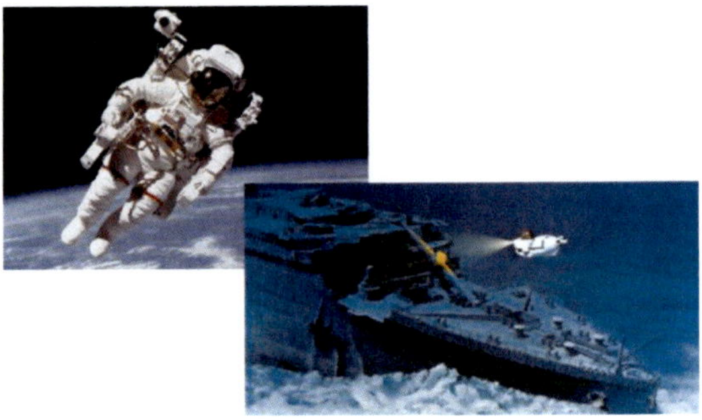

Figure 1. The achievements of modern technology are truly impressive.

It concerns the development of technology working for medicine as well. Not only better and better diagnostic systems (Figure 2) but numerous devices supporting the treatment process are created (Figure 3). It could seem that the situation is very good.

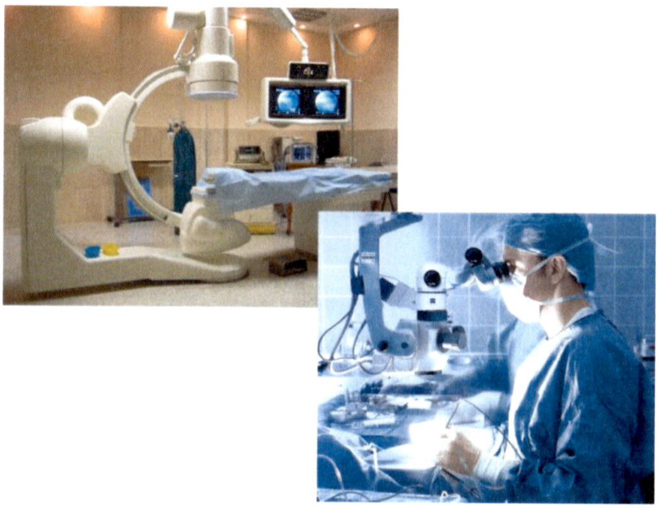

Figure 2. There has been a huge improvement in terms of technical devices created for the purpose of medical diagnosis.

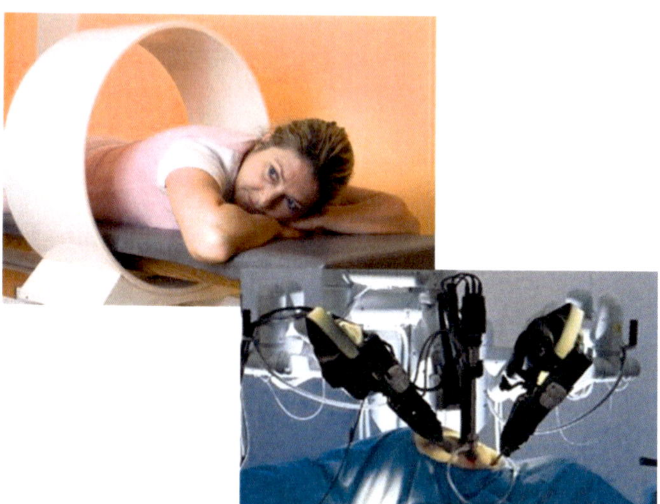

Figure 3. There are a number of technical devices supporting therapy.

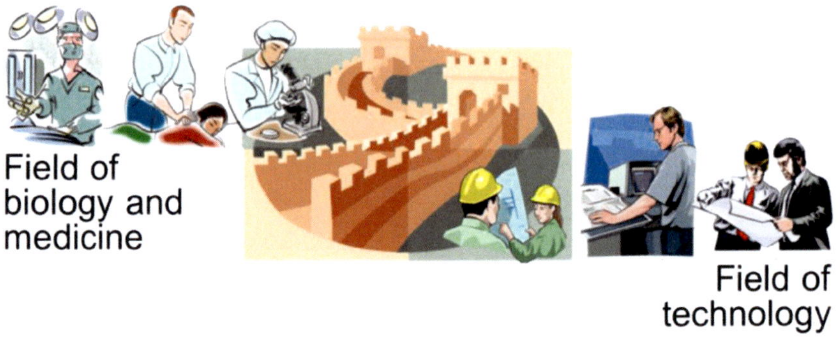

Figure 4. A symbolic representation of the differences between the fields of biology and technology as "wall."

However, in reality, the transfer of scientific ideas between the field of biology and the field of technology is still much impeded. And it does not come out of someone's bad will. The simple truth is that the huge progress of biology and medicine on the one hand and the development of technology on the other led to the situation that a peculiar mental "wall" (Figure 4) has grown between the two fields. It is the wall of different methodology and different developmental traditions as well as a hermetic, different terminology. We will try to show that the new branch of science, which biocybernetics is, may help medical doctors and technicians to communicate "discounting the differences," despite that "wall."

I will quote examples from the field of medicine as being the creator of the Biomedical Engineering study I seem to know something about it, yet, of course, not as much as professional medical doctors. That is why, as an example of the existence of that "wall" I will present the blood pressure stabilization system. Blood pressure stability might be considered from both the point of view of medicine and biology. As it is widely known, each more complex organism developed a system of blood pressure, thanks to which blood carrying oxygen and nutrients reaches all organs and tissues ensuring beneficial life conditions for cells creating them. That blood must have stable pressure (adjusted to the needs). Nature created a lot of mechanisms (neural and hormonal) which are used to achieve that goal. As the next system, let us consider the pressure stabilization system in technical installations. It is also necessary since technical systems are used to transfer various fluids. The water pipeline reaching houses, hydraulic brakes in cars, reactors in a chemical plant are a few examples of such systems through which pressurized fluids have to flow. That pressure must be stabilized so engineers found out a variety of devices serving that goal. Both examples concern the same problem, i.e., the system ensuring pressure stability. However biologists on the one hand and engineers on the other present the object of their interest in such a different way that transferring the knowledge from one field to the other is practically impossible. It is a pity because such a diffusion of knowledge from one field to the other might be very beneficial. If hematologists and cardiologists dealing with blood pressure stabilization knew the methods which are used by engineers in their regulatory systems, they might be able to improve their methods of diagnostics and therapy. And the other way round, if plumbers knew what kind of clever systems of pressure control "were invented" by biology and how they have been perfected for millions of years of evolution, they would be able to build new more effective regulators avoiding costly research looking for an optimal structure by trial and error methods. However, specialists of both mentioned parties may understand and use only their part of knowledge and the part which is on the other side is "black magic" for them. The above is the example of how the "wall" depicted in Figure 4 functions.

How to Overturn that Difficulty?

It is not possible (or sensible) for engineers to learn physiology or for doctors to learn the secrets of mechanics. Nevertheless it is possible to suggest such a description of the considered systems and processes, which will match both biological phenomena and technical devices. What is more, the methods of using that description will be equally easy for doctors as for engineers, and presenting particular issues using such a description biological subjects will become comprehensible for technicians and technical constructions will be understandable for biologists. Biocybernetics offers such ways of description and that is why it can be used as a peculiar "bridge" allowing for overcoming the differences dividing technology from biology and medicine. Due to that it is possible to cross the "wall" dividing the mentioned fields (Figure 5).

How is it Possible to Achieve That Effect?

The Key to Success is Abstraction. Let us look at Figure 6

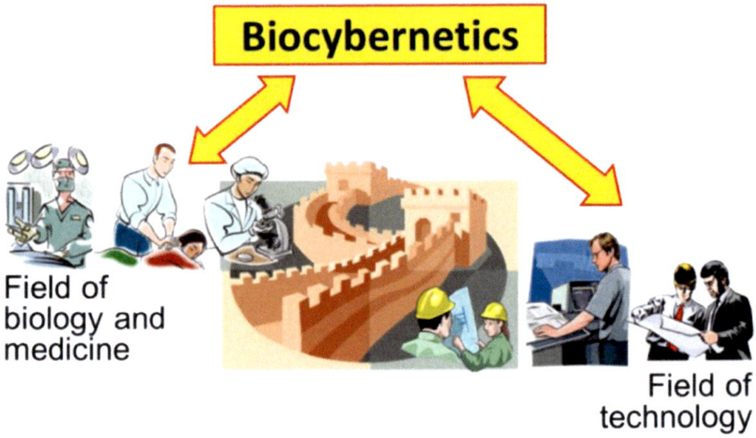

Figure 5. The role of biocybernetics as an element permitting overcome the differences separating the field of biology and medicine and the field of technology.

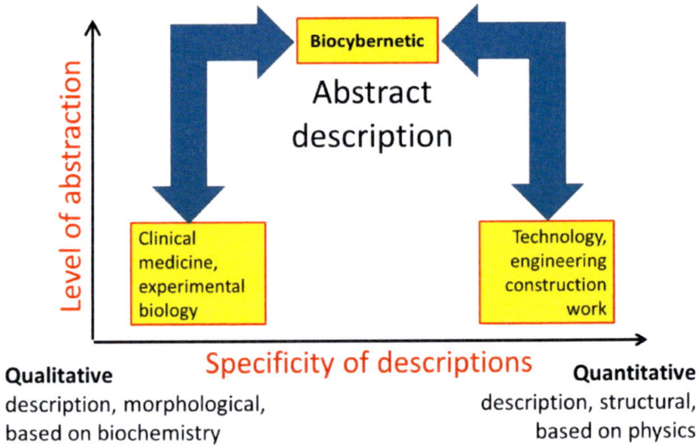

Figure 6. Thanks to the high level of abstraction the description created on the basis of biocybernetics can fit both to biology, as well as technology.

The figure depicts that biology (especially experimental biology) and medicine (mainly clinical medicine) are the fields of very down to earth activities characterized by a very low level of abstraction. On the other hand, technology together with construction, engineering and technical work is an area of very concrete activities featuring a low level of abstraction as well. With those particular activities the characteristics of both biological and technical system descriptions plays an important role. That characteristic causes difficulties while trying to transfer biological discoveries into technical creativity areas and fundamentally hinders creating technical solutions for biological and medical needs. However, when you release particular descriptions (both biological and technical) from details which decide upon that characteristics and create a description with a high level of abstraction, which is offered by biocybernetics, then the points of view of medical doctors and technicians may be reconciled. Mutual agreement will be possible and there will be an inspiring transfer of ideas, a new value resulting from biological-technical synergy will be created giving an effect of progress both in biology and in technology.

A high level of abstraction of biocybernetic descriptions, mentioned above as a way of transferring information from the field of biology to the field technology (and the other way round) may also be used as a favorable factor for developing both medicine and biology themselves. It happens from time to time, that developing practical activities within clinical medicine or experimental biology is hindered by various obstacles (Figure 7).

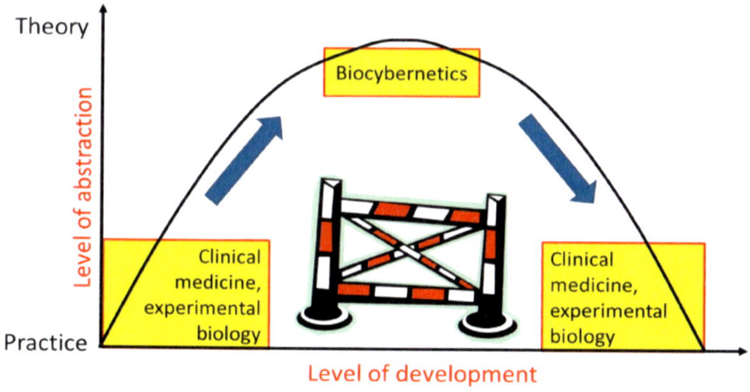

Figure 7. Biocybernetics as a way of overcoming obstacles to the development of biology and medicine.

In such cases the obstacles may be overcome by shifting from clear practice to a more abstract look at the issues under question. And also in such a situation referring to a biocybernetic theory may allow for overcoming the practical obstacle and favor obtaining new solutions perfecting the practice. A frequent ingredient of such new solutions may not only be a better technical equipment of medicine obtained due to biomedical engineering but medical procedures might be perfected as well when you look at them from the "bird eye view."

How can the "Bird Eye View" be Achieved in Practice?

One should tear apart from unimportant details and bring the core of matter to the surface. Build a biocybernetic model. In science, e.g., in chemistry, creating an abstract model is usually preceded by experimentation (Figure 8).

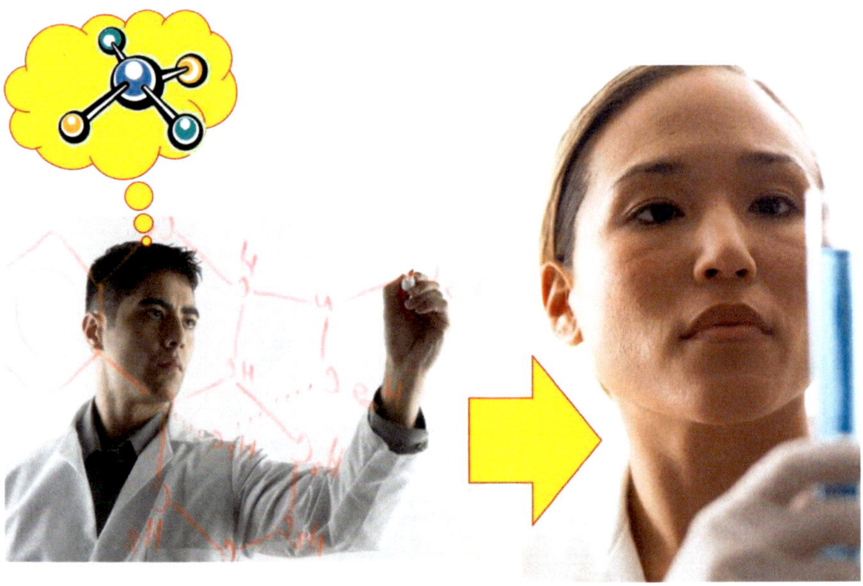

Figure 8. When creating new chemical compounds (e.g., new drugs) is typically first formed an abstract model of the desired molecule, and then carried out the synthesis and examined the properties of the new compound.

Creating an abstract model may help in scientific discoveries or in a correct interpretation of that information which is supplied by empirical experiments. It can be observed on the basis of development in astronomy, especially on the knowledge on the structure of the Solar System, i.e., a collection of planets our Earth belongs to as well. Basing on simple observation they were the ancient astronomers who discovered that among stationary stars there are five celestial bodies in the sky which move in a strange and interesting way. They called those bodies "planets" as the word "planet" means a wanderer in Greek. The planets were given names: Mercury, Venus, Mars, Jove (Jupiter) and Saturn. For over one thousand years it was all the astronomical knowledge that people had. However, later Nicolaus Copernicus created a theory (speculative, as it was not based on experiment but on reasoning) according to which the Earth became the sixth planet of the Solar System. The next planet of the System was impossible to discover with the naked eye so it was noticed by William Herschel only when the astronomer used an appropriate research tool (the telescope). But those might have been years that the last planet of the Solar System (Neptune) might have been looked for using most powerful telescopes as it is extremely difficult to notice it since it is not a star but a planet. It was discovered, however, by Urban Le Verrier, who used a mathematical model of all known planets of the Solar System and discovered that the model gives results that do not fall into place with observations. The only explanation was putting another, unknown planet into the model and Le Verrier showed where it should be. When he notified the astronomical observatory in Berlin about his discovery (theoretical, made only via a model), Johann Gottfried Galle discovered the planet within a quarter of an hour. As it appeared the planet had been observed for hundreds of years by throngs of astronomers (the first one to notice Neptune by his telescope was Galileo) not knowing what they had observed in fact.

That short story of astronomical discoveries may lead to drawing the following conclusions: On a certain stage of getting to know the Nature, knowledge comes mainly from observation. Subsequently, that knowledge may be enriched referring to speculative theories (in biology the counterpart of Copernicus' theory may be Darwin's theory). On a certain stage the progress of research is guaranteed by the continually perfected research equipment. But when the enumerated above sources deplete, progress may be ensured mainly by a model which enables to foresee empirical discoveries before they are made and which allows to understand the meaning of the empirical discovery, the interpretation of which might not be easy in the case of really important discoveries.

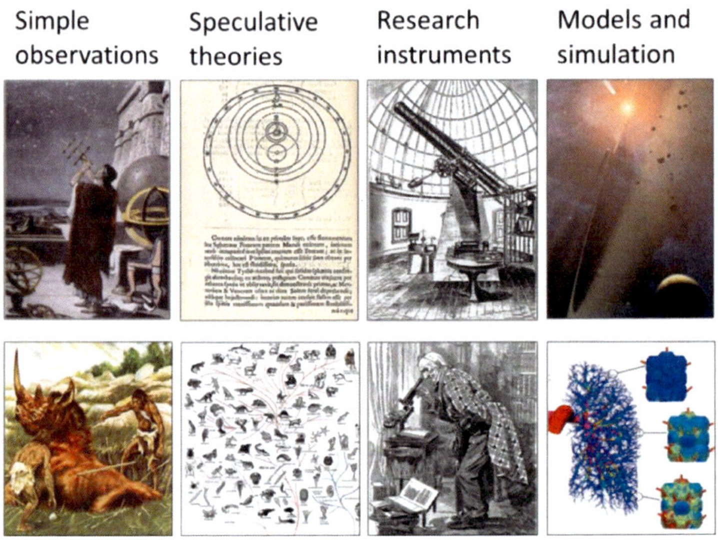

Figure 9. Parallelism stages of development of biological knowledge with respect to the discussed in the text development of astronomical knowledge.

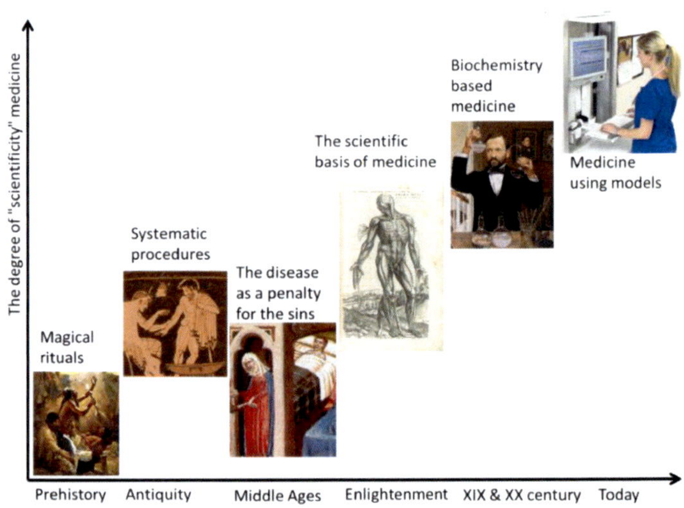

Figure 10. The history of the development of medicine exposing the role of biocybernetic models in modern medicine.

The story told above concerned astronomy, but one may easily show a similar sequence of discoveries which were made on particular stages of medical and biological knowledge development with the end of the sequence showing an inspiring and initiating role of models in biology, and, of course, I mean biocybernetic models. This was shown in Figure 9 depicting the concurrency of biological knowledge development in comparison to the astronomical knowledge mentioned above.

The role of biocybernetic models in the development of medicine is depicted in Figure 10. It shows how the way of looking at and understanding health and disease influenced the rate of scholarship (and the rate of efficiency) of medical activities. In the prehistoric period people believed that illness was caused by magical factors (bad charms thrown by people, presence of demons, etc.), so while treating people magic practice was used as well (use of drums, tribal dances and songs, using incense etc.). Rational ancient civilization led to a systematization of treatment procedures, with the choice of procedures dictated by empirical knowledge and not theories on the cause and result processes.

Although during the Middle Ages numerous hospitals subordinated to the duty of mercy and care of the sufferers originated but the scientific level of medical care receded in comparison to the knowledge which was presented by ancient medics as the domineering belief was that a disease was a punishment for sins and one should not resist it. The turnover within the field (just like in lots of other) was brought by the Enlightenment period when constructing scientific basis of medicine through learning anatomy first (post-mortem examinations became permitted) followed by physiology. That scientific foundation has been used by medicine until today.

A triumphant march of biochemistry followed. Exceptionally well recognized biochemical processes connected to metabolism and cells, tissues and whole organs functioning caused that the human organism began to be perceived as a particular chemical reactor (Figure 11). A natural consequence of such an optics was the so far practiced estimation of the state of the organism by taking and chemical analysis of samples, blood and other body fluids, urine and other excrements, cells and tissues sampled during biopsy, etc. It is assumed that finding out an incorrect composition of those samples is an important clue in the reasoning aiming at defining the character of the disease and the way of treating it.

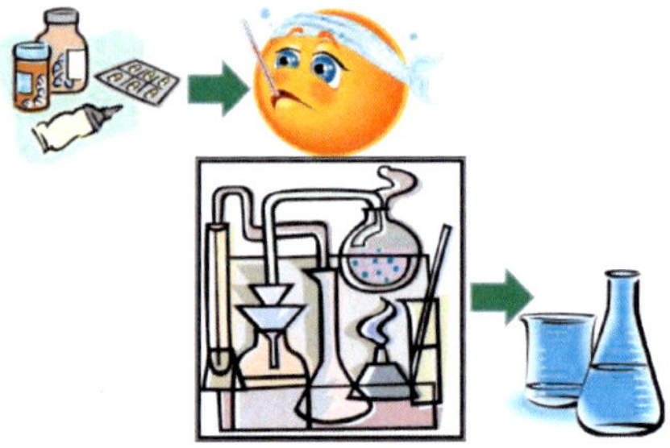

Figure 11. The sick man's body treated as chemical reactor.

Treatment itself is strongly based on biochemical basis as we use numerous pharmaceutical products (tablets, injections, suppositories, etc.) working more or less according to the following cognitive scheme: if the organism is a chemical reactor and something is wrong with it, one must add something to the reactor to supply the missing ingredients or neutralize the ingredients which are abundant. That is how our medical diagnostics and therapy have looked until today. On the other hand, the medicine of tomorrow will be strongly based upon the analysis of all cause and result processes which take place in a living organism. One must, of course, take into consideration biochemical processes as no one wants to negate their important role in all health and disease matters but one should consider physical processes as well since human organism is also a very complicated and easily broken machine (Figure 12), not forgetting about information processes which play the check-up and controlling parts in relation to all other discussed processes.

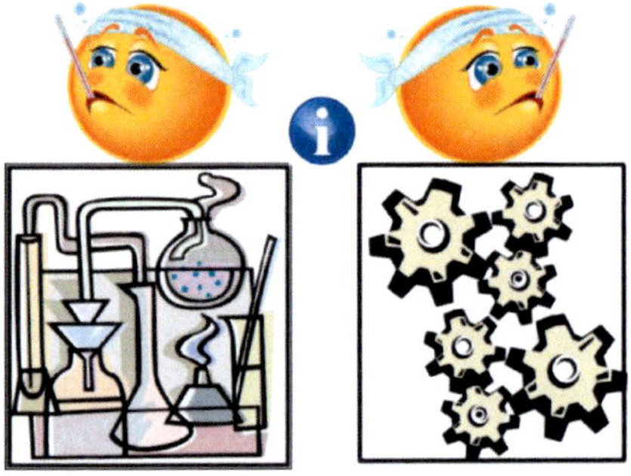

Figure 12. A look at the human body through the prism of chemical processes, physical mechanisms and information as a control factor .

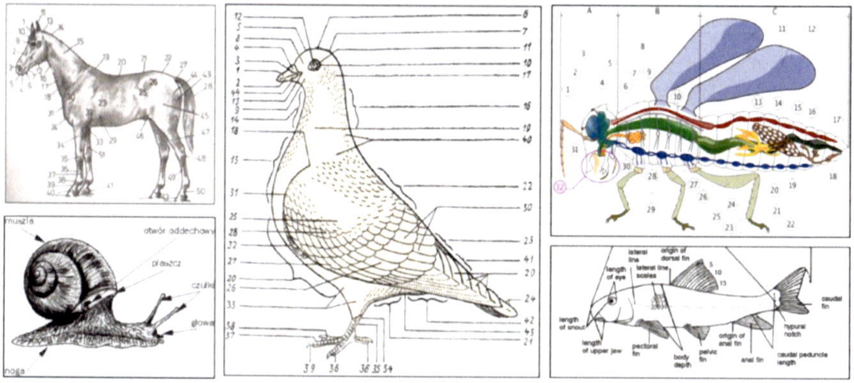

Figure 13. Examples of the diversity of the animal world.

To take control over the growing complexity of human organism descriptions in those three above mentioned perspectives one needs biocybernetic models. Their power is held in the possibility of using abstraction as a factor remarkably reducing the complexity of the considered problems. I will illustrate that by an attempt of constructing an abstract model of an animal. Not a horse, a snail or a pigeon but a "generalized animal," so general that the model will include a human organism model. How to do it if we estimate that there are currently about 8.7 million species out of which there about 1.2 million which are exactly described? After all each animal has its special characteristics and each of them is different from another. Figure 13 depicts various animals. One can see how much they differ. Having so much detailed information about each species of animals it seems it is practically impossible to give any general opinion about all animals. However, building on cybernetics, one can try to do it.

To gain a model of a "general animal" which will describe all those countless creatures' one must reject detailed information about them. One must disregard them. Thanks to such abstraction we will learn what is common for all animals and thus which is the most important feature. The first attempt for such an abstraction is depicted in Figure 14. The figure shows two abstract (i.e., deprived of any detailed features) objects: the considered **animal** and the **environment**. Let us notice that both objects in Figure 14 are represented by blocks, which have nothing to do with their real shapes. The oval block certainly does not resemble the body of any animal, while the rectangle does not look like any real environment. The relationship between the blocks and real objects has only an arbitrary character and that is why the flow chart is an example of a formal model which is used in biocybernetics all the time.

We will begin to fill the interior of the block representing the abstract animal with subsequent systems ensuring the realization of functions which each animal must fulfill. The first of them is **activity**. The form of activity may vary but the presence of activity allows for differentiation of each living creature from any piece of non-living matter. To show activity one must possess a possibility of movement. And again there is a vast variety of organs and systems ensuring movement to animals. Water animals move in another way as land animals, which is still different from flying creatures. But a movement system in this or that form is present with all of them, which is illustrated by Figure 15.

Activity should be purposeful, i.e., connected to the **perception** of the state of the environment. Thanks to the environment state perception one may localize food and notice the approaching danger (a predator which wants to treat our model animal as his meal). Impulses coming from the environment allow for finding a sexual partner and a safe hideout to survive the period of lowered activity. That is why the animal must possess a perception system in order to receive those impulses and interpret them correctly. For the perception system to bring positive effects it must be connected to an earlier introduced movement system, since only then the animal will be able to capture the noticed food effectively, successfully avoid the observed threats and skillfully join its sexual partner. Due to this a **nervous system** is needed to carry information from the perception system to the movement system.

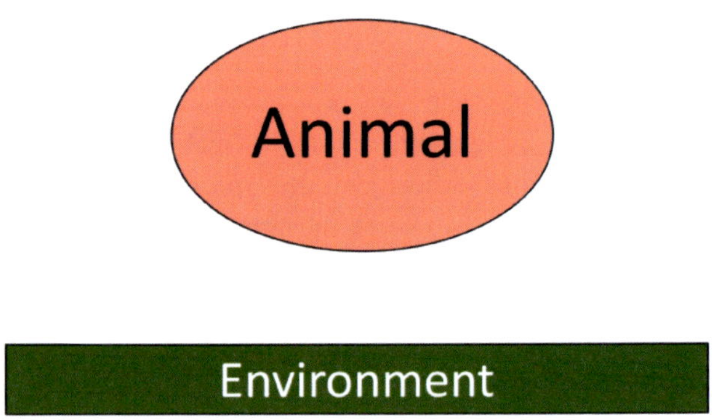

Figure 14. Beginning of creating of the abstract animal model.

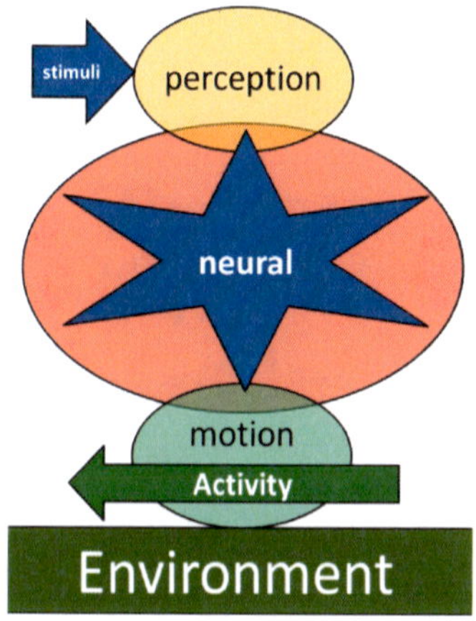

Figure 15. Animal model additionally equipped with systems: perceptual and nervous.

However, it is not only information that an animal lives on. Energy is needed to show its activity and nutritional substances are needed to develop and potentially repair its body. That is why each animal must draw food and oxygen from its environment (for energy processes which have an aerobic character in most animals) and excrete unused parts of food and carbon dioxide. Our animal model must be equipped additionally with digestive and respiratory systems together with a circulatory system which will supply food and oxygen to all tissues and organs of the body and dispose of carbon dioxide created in metabolic processes, which was depicted in Figure 16.

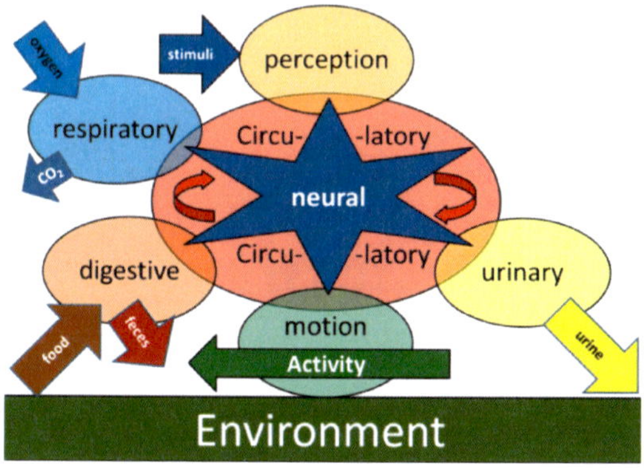

Figure 16. Animal model which takes into account energetic processes.

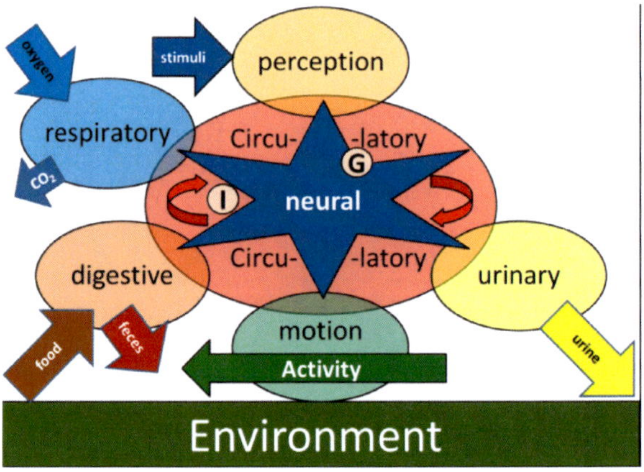

Figure 17. The next stage of enrichment animal model by the immune system and glands.

Metabolism causes creating (apart from carbon dioxide) other waste products as well, which must be disposed of by the urinary system while in the circulatory system there are also elements of the organism protection against various microbiological threats (the role is played by the immunological system depicted in Figure 17 by the symbol "I") and regulatory elements with a prolonged time of activity and with a more general character than neural controlling. That last role is played by hormones, the source of which is the system of endocrine glands, marked by the symbol "G").

Finally the considered model of an animal must be equipped with a genital system thanks to which the animal will be able to proliferate and ensure species survival despite a limited life span of each specimen (Figure 18).

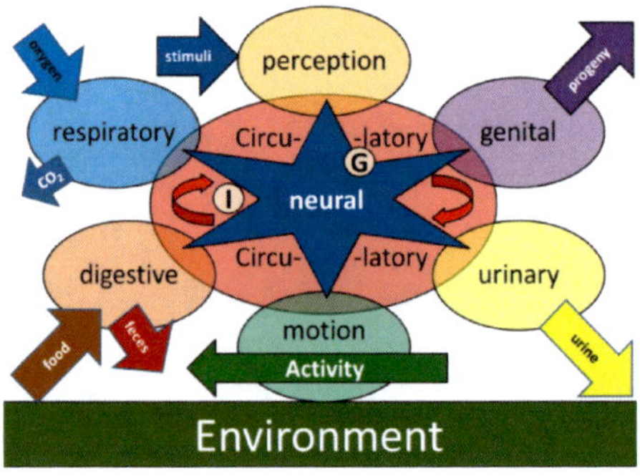

Figure 18. The final structure of the animal model.

Obviously the way of building a model of an animal presented above contains a lot of simplifications (e.g., exocrine glands were not taken into account) but my point was to signal the direction of activities undertaken by biocyberneticians and not to go into details.

The construction and use of a biocybernetic model is a process including a few stages. At the beginning as big as possible reserve of biological knowledge is collected on the modeled biological system. The source of that knowledge may be laboratory tests (in vitro), experiments on animals (in vivo), clinical observations on people and various statistical data. That knowledge must then be properly selected (to make it concern the considered issues and not introduce side subjects) and analyzed in detail by experts (not to contain false, incomplete or untypical information). The discussed introductory activities are depicted in Figure 19.

Then the data derived from the adequately analyzed biological observations undergoes formalization as a result of which a mathematical model is created. It is common for complex biological systems that their biocybernetic models are also complicated so their direct interpretation may be impossible. But having a model in a mathematical form one may build a computer program performing any needed calculations based on the formulae of that mathematical model relatively easily. Such a program is usually called a simulation program and the research run by its means is called simulation research. That simulation research is a key component of each biocybernetician's work so we can concentrate on what kind of research that is and what it is run for.

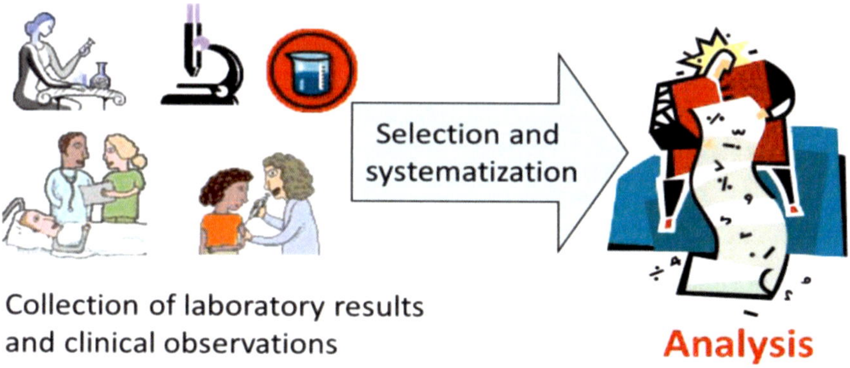

Figure 19. The beginning of the construction process of biocybernetic model.

A computer program containing a mathematical description of a biocybernetic model allows, by calculations, to simulate various situations, in which the biological object described by the model may be found. Behavior of such a computer simulated object may be observed closely as it is possible to check each number on the computer. Initially, simulation experiments are run in such a way as to reproduce the situations, in which the modeled biological object was observed and its behavior is known exactly. If the simulation model does not reproduce that known behavior one must return to mathematical formalization and look for a better mathematical model. Of course if the experiments checking the correctness of the model's work give positive results, one is able to attempt some new, earlier unknown facts by means of the checked model. Therefore situations and circumstances, which have never been used while testing the model empirically, are created in the model (by numerical methods). In such a case, observing the results of the computer simulation one can gain new information and new facts enriching the knowledge on the researched (modeled) object. Such a way of biocybernetic attainment of new knowledge on objects and biological processes has already gained big respect among researchers and is sometimes called an "*experiment in compute*" to resemble traditionally held biological experiments on tissues separated from organisms, called an "*experiment in vitro*" and experiments on animals called an "*experiment in vivo*." The results of simulation experiments must obviously undergo an analysis to draw all possible conclusions, which is depicted in Figure 20.

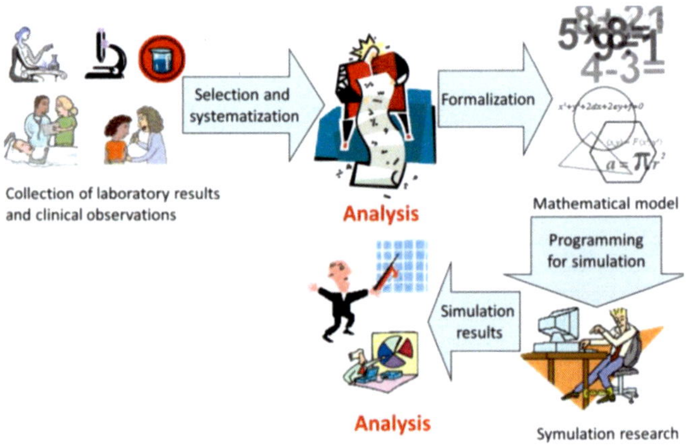

Figure 20. The transition from biological knowledge into mathematical model and computer simulation.

The results received from a computer simulation of a biocybernetic model may contain most valuable scientific discoveries, yet one must verify them. Only the result verified on a real biological object (that is the one that was repeated in a laboratory test or confirmed by clinical observation) has a scientific or/and practical value. That is why to run a fully successful research using a biocybernetic model it is necessary to gain a positive empirical confirmation of its results, thanks to which (with a positive result of the mentioned verification) the practical zone may be substantially enriched. It is worth noticing that such empirical research of a biological object in order to confirm (or falsify) the results achieved before in the way of computer simulation is much more effective than running biological experiments "in the dark" not knowing what a researcher will get. In such a case the simulation model props the researcher what and where to look, which results to expect and how to interpret them. Similarly to the mentioned above story of Neptune discovery, the last planet of the Solar System which was possible to discover as its existence together with its location had been foreseen earlier by means of a model. In biology such a method of result anticipation before running experiments has not been widely used yet, but the development of biocybernetics guides us towards such solutions so the situation will certainly change radically in the future.

A closed cycle of research finished with a positive verification of computer simulation is shown in Figure 21.

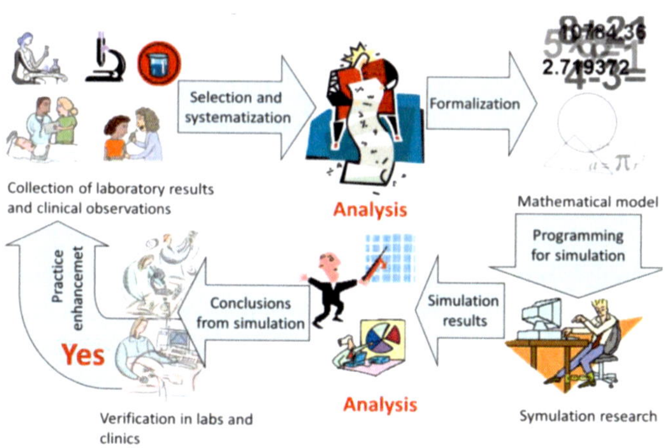

Figure 21. A complete cycle of research aimed at obtaining new useful practical results based on biocybernetic modeling.

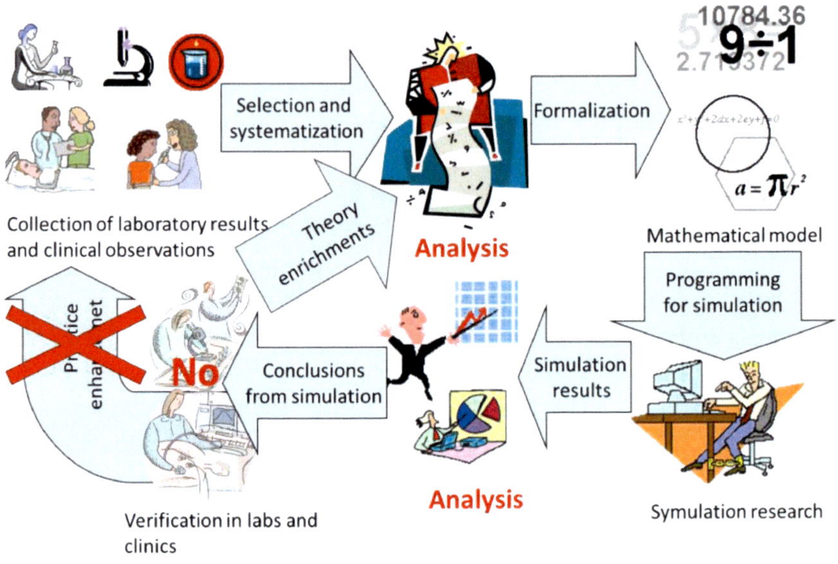

Figure 22. The result of biocybernetic modeling in the form of modification of widely accepted theory.

Interestingly enough, an unsuccessful empirical verification of a result achieved previously by means of a simulation based upon a biocybernetic model may, unexpectedly, have a positive value. It is implied by the fact that the whole part of the schematic diagram shown in Figure 22, beginning with formalization of biomedical data results and ending with the analysis of simulation results is under strong control within correctness and accuracy of the reasoning, within the adequacy of used methods and achieved test results. Within that area no errors should appear. If the final result is erroneous, the only explanation is that biological data was badly interpreted on the stage of its analysis. In other words our theory (biological) on how the considered biological system is built, how it functions and what the main conditions of its activity is, were mistaken. In other words it only seemed to us that we know and understand that biological system but when we tried to base upon that knowledge and used the preconceived notions based upon our imagination that we understand that system we reached a contradiction (the model did not confirm the conclusions drawn from that reasoning). Theory did not withstand confrontation with practice. And if it is like that the theory must be changed! We know this kind of result of modeling various systems (physical, technical, social, economic) from practice. It has often happened in the history of science that someone gifted with a high level of articulateness and possessing great authority suggested some theory and no potential critic was able to defy the elaborate rhetorical argument nor even dared to undermine the opinion of the expert given such common trust. However, computers have the feature that they are insensitive to the influence of arguments and do not take into consideration whose ideas they defy. For a computer only logic and exact calculation have meaning. And an elaborate theory may collapse. Of course, the result is less impressive than adding a new, previously unknown scientific discovery. Nevertheless it is useful as building upon a false theory may be very dangerous.

Concluding this chapter one must claim that biocybernetics is still not a commonly used method supplementing traditional research methods in biology and medicine but it has a chance to become a commonly used procedure and I strongly believe that it will be another mechanism propelling progress in biology and medicine, especially within carcinogenesis and cancer treatment.

References

[1] Calzone, L; Fages, F; Soliman; S. BIOCHAM: an environment for modeling biological systems and formalizing experimental knowledge, *Bioinformatics*, 2015, 22(14), 1805-1807

[2] Guigen, Zhang. (2015). Computational Bioengineering. CRC Press

[3] Haefner, JW. (2005). Modeling Biological Systems: Principles and Applications, Springer Science & Business Media.

[4] Tadeusiewicz, R. (2013). Biocybernetics - Methodological Fundamentals for Biomedical Engineering [In Polish: Biocybernetyka – Metodologiczne podstawy dla inżynierii biomedycznej], PWN, Warszawa.

[5] Tadeusiewicz, R; Jaworek, J; Kańtoch, E; Miller, J; Pięciak, T; Przybyło, J. (2012). Introduction to modeling of biological systems and their simulation in MATLAB environment [In Polish: Wprowadzenie do modelowania systemów biologicznych oraz ich symulacji w środowisku MATLAB], UMCS Lublin.

INDEX

C

D

J

K

L

M

N

O

P

Q

R

S

W

Z